PRAISE FOR *SACRED COW*

"Diana and Robb have answered the burning question about meat. *Sacred Cow* proves 'It's not the COW, it's the HOW.' The answer to our broken food system is not no meat, it's better meat. If you are concerned about red meat's impact on your health and the planet, this book is for you."

—Mark Hyman, MD, Cleveland Clinic Center for Functional Medicine

"Public perception surrounding the environmental impacts of red meat is at the center of our food debates, and Diana and Robb have precisely and approachably laid out the science on how grazing animals are critical to the future of sustainable agriculture. They also definitively refute the claims that meat is unhealthy and make a convincing case that eating meat can be done in an ethical manner. I highly recommend *Sacred Cow* for anyone who eats."

—Mark Sisson, *New York Times* bestselling author of *The Keto Reset Diet* and founder of Primal Kitchen foods

"Humans have been eating meat for at least 2.6 million years, and it has played a critical role in our evolution. In this important book, Diana Rodgers and Robb Wolf use the most recent scientific evidence to make the nutritional, environmental, and ethical case for better meat—and to debunk increasingly common myths and misunderstandings about the role of animal products in our diet."

—Chris Kresser, *New York Times* bestselling author of *The Paleo Cure* and *Unconventional Medicine*

"*Sacred Cow: The Case for Better Meat* is a comprehensive, well documented treatise that provides us with all the scientific data we need to make informed choices about how to eat that will benefit BOTH ourselves and our planet!"

—Frederick Kirschenmann, PhD, Distinguished Fellow at the Leopold Center for Sustainable Agriculture at Iowa State University

"Abandoning animal agriculture might well be the greatest mistake humanity could ever make. Today's science cannot give definitive answers to the complex questions of human nutrition and ecological integrity. However, the scientific evidence indicting animal agriculture is weak, and evidence defending animal-based foods and farm animals as essential for human health and agricultural sustainability is strong—as clearly documented in *Sacred Cow*. Perhaps the most important truth in this well-written, highly readable book is that the continuation of life depends on death: 'We are all part of a food web and the inevitable cycle of life, which includes death.'"

—John Ikerd, PhD, professor emeritus of agricultural economics at the University of Missouri

"The current war against meat eaters and livestock farmers promises ethical, ecological, and health benefits from fake lab meat and plant-only diets. *Sacred Cow* debunks every utopian promise with precision missiles from science and a deep understanding of how life and the planet actually work."

—Joel Salatin, owner of Polyface Farm and editor of *The Stockman Grass Farmer*

"The shift in agriculture, from one based on biology to one based on chemistry, and the resulting shift in our diets from whole foods to highly processed foods have resulted in nutrition-related disease, obesity, and environmental destruction. Diana and Robb fully understand the problem and the solution: we must change our diets and regenerate our soils, and well-managed grazing animals are critical to this transition."

—Allan Savory, president of Savory Institute and chairman of the Africa Center for Holistic Management

"So much of the confusion about creating a sustainable future is based on a misunderstanding of ecology, evolution, and our place within the natural world. Much of our confusion has to do with our increasing separation from nature, especially how our food is produced. This book clearly explains how it all fits together, and how the interwoven evolution of ruminants, grasslands, and homo sapiens is not something to be left in the past, but to be celebrated and reclaimed."

—Mark A. Ritchie, PhD, executive director of the International Sustainable Development Studies Institute

"I once stopped eating meat because I thought it would keep me free of disease, release the world's food animals from incomprehensible suffering, and save the planet from destruction. Twelve cavities, two root canals, and an assortment of anxiety disorders later, I realized this choice had come at the expense of my own health. If I had known about a healthier way to eat meat, one that respects animals and can support the health of the planet, I may have saved my health a lot of trouble. If only I'd have had access to *Sacred Cow*! Diana and Robb have written a tour de force making the case that meat can be good for our bodies, the animals, and the earth. *Sacred Cow* is the antidote to miserably meatless mondays and impossibly impotent impossible burgers. The cure is an ethical approach to eating animals, giving them their rightful place in our ecology."

—Chris Masterjohn, PhD, former assistant professor of Health and Nutrition Sciences at Brooklyn College

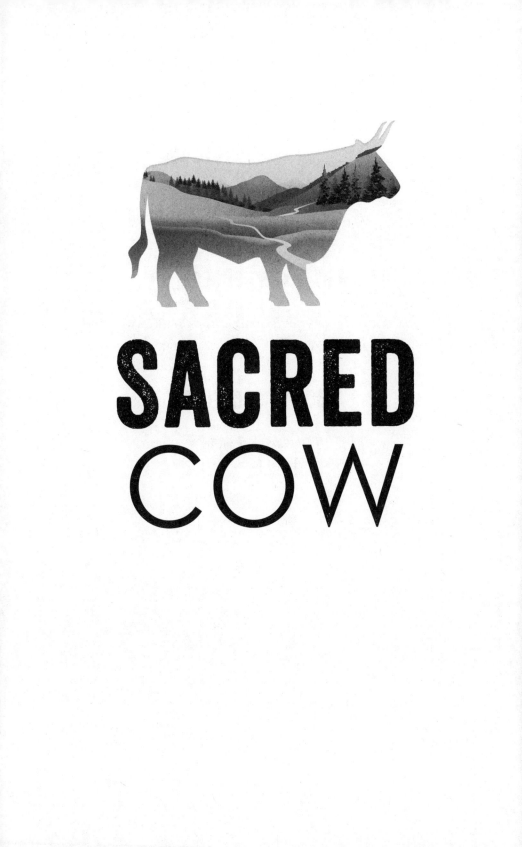

SACRED
COW

ALSO BY DIANA RODGERS, RD

Paleo Lunches and Breakfasts on the Go
The Homegrown Paleo Cookbook

ALSO BY ROBB WOLF

The Paleo Solution
Wired to Eat

SACRED COW

THE CASE FOR (BETTER) MEAT

DIANA RODGERS, RD
ROBB WOLF

BenBella Books, Inc.
Dallas, TX

Sacred Cow copyright © 2020 by Diana Rodgers and Robert Wolf

Interior graphics by James Cooper (ONIC Design), unless otherwise credited.

BenBella Books, Inc.
10440 N. Central Expressway, Suite 800
Dallas, TX 75231
www.benbellabooks.com
Send feedback to feedback@benbellabooks.com

BenBella is a federally registered trademark.

Printed in the United States of America
10 9 8 7 6 5 4 3 2 1

Library of Congress Control Number: 2020001636
ISBN 9781948836913 (hardcover)
ISBN 9781950665112 (electronic)

Editing by Claire Schulz
Copyediting by Miki Alexandra Caputo
Proofreading by Lisa Story and Cape Cod Compositors, Inc.
Indexing by Amy Murphy
Text design and composition by Aaron Edmiston
Cover design by Emily Weigel and James Cooper
Cover photo © Shutterstock / jagoda (landscape) and © Dreamstime / Gpgroup (bull)
Printed by Lake Book Manufacturing

Distributed to the trade by Two Rivers Distribution, an Ingram brand
www.tworiversdistribution.com

Special discounts for bulk sales are available.
Please contact bulkorders@benbellabooks.com.

*For our children. May they steward this world
better than those who came before them.*

CONTENTS

PART I: THE NUTRITIONAL CASE FOR (BETTER) MEAT

PART II: THE ENVIRONMENTAL CASE FOR (BETTER) MEAT

PART III: THE ETHICAL CASE FOR (BETTER) MEAT

PART IV: WHAT WE CAN DO

For more information on the issues described in this book and the *Sacred Cow* documentary film, please visit Sacredcow.info.

INTRODUCTION

At our grocery stores and dinner tables, even the most thought-
ful consumers are overwhelmed when choosing how to eat
right—especially when it comes to meat.

It's an ethical, environmental, and nutritional conundrum. We
want a food system that is sustainable and provides us with fantastic
nutrition. Most of us want to follow the noble principle of doing
least harm. And when we're confronted with the legitimate horrors
of the modern industrial food system, and a flood of contradictory
messages coming from mainstream health experts and the media,
many have resolved the quandary by reducing the amount of meat
they eat or cutting it out entirely. Surely a meat-free diet is the only
approach that can be environmentally sustainable for the long haul,
and we've heard it's better for us anyway.

The notion that meat is unhealthy and bad for the environment
is, in some circles, "settled science." The arguments are simple,
powerful, and compelling: meat, they say, causes cancer, heart disease, and diabetes and is disproportionately damaging to the environment. These appealingly unambiguous "elevator pitch" claims
get repeated by Hollywood stars, tech moguls, ideological groups,
food companies.

Yet when we dig deeper, we discover nuances and details that
can't be captured in sound bites or memes. It's a complex story that

spans physics, chemistry, biology, and ecology (to say nothing of psychology and the thorny topic of economics). It's become quite clear to us we're being told a story about what's best for our bodies and the planet. And that story may at best be inaccurate and at worst an existential threat. In a nutshell, the prejudice that meat is bad for health and the environment and that eating it is a morally objectionable practice has effectively become a "sacred cow." The *Concise Oxford English Dictionary* defines the term thus:

> **Sacred cow: an idea, custom, or institution held, especially unreasonably, to be above criticism.**

What is sold as sustainable, ethical, and healthy is a food system without animals, or at least one that involves substantially less meat than our current levels of consumption. These notions are accepted largely as fact. But the evidence—although it's difficult to unpack—is clearly not consistent with these ideas.

WHO ARE WE AND WHY ARE WE WRITING THIS BOOK NOW?

Diana is a registered dietitian with a clinical practice helping people recover their health through real food. Her blog, *Sustainable Dish*, started as a healthy, locally sourced recipe site but has grown into a much deeper dive into food systems. She has spent the last eighteen years living on a working organic farm that grows vegetables and raises pasture-based meat. She met Robb in 2011 after reading his book *The Paleo Solution*, which has sold nearly a million copies.

Trained as a research biochemist, Robb discovered that the optimal human diet is one that most closely mimics our ancestral way of eating, before the invention of ultraprocessed foods.

Both of us have dealt with severe digestive issues, have minds that question everything, and are always looking to find the truth behind commonly held beliefs. In addition to our firsthand experience with food production and our deep backgrounds in science, we've read many books, interviewed experts, and have attended a remarkable number of conferences on agriculture. When we met, we quickly bonded over our interest not only in optimal human health but in discovering which food production methods were best from a sustainability perspective. For various reasons, the majority of health experts seem to have little, if any, firsthand knowledge or formal education in food production and sustainability. (When Diana was in her graduate nutrition program, the only class on food procurement focused solely on how to obtain food service commodities at the lowest price—no thought was given to where and how that food was actually grown.) And, on the other side, most agriculture and environmental experts tend not to consider optimal human nutritional needs in their arguments. Everyone seems to be tackling "the future of food" from their individual silos, with little knowledge or appreciation of the system as a whole. So, the intersection of this Venn diagram is something not many have explored.

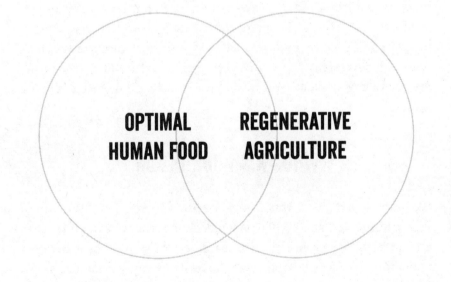

Where do they overlap? To us, it makes perfect sense that we should strive for a diet that closely mimics what humans have evolved to eat and implement agricultural systems that follow nature as much as possible. In this book we'll walk you through how we came to these conclusions.

We have been talking about the ideas in this book for many years (Robb's first public discussion on the ethical, health, and environmental considerations of a meat-inclusive food system was in 2006). But the amount of work required to intelligently unpack these complex arguments seemed daunting—and it still was even when we wrote this book, to be honest!

And yet, now is the time to have this discussion. The debate is picking up momentum in the food world; folks are giving more and more attention to finding a diet that will both feed a growing population and preserve the planet.

Both of us have spent an enormous amount of time studying this topic and attempting to poke holes in not just *our* conclusions but the conclusions of the source material we cite throughout this work. Through our research, what we've discovered is that, contrary to the popular narrative, red meat is one of the most nutrient-dense foods available; indeed, the extent of access to nutrient-dense animal products such as meat is one of the greatest distinguishers between the poor and wealthy in developed or developing countries. Perhaps more controversially, when raised properly, cattle and other grazers may be one of our most promising tools toward mitigating climate change.

WHO THIS BOOK IS FOR

We want to be clear: this book is not "anti-vegan." Oftentimes, strong feelings come into play when deciding what to eat, and there's a large body of psychological research establishing that it's almost impossible to sway people who have made emotional decisions. However, we feel that with a complete understanding of the nutritional and environmental argument *for* better meat a more nuanced ethical discussion can begin to take place.

In our increasingly polarized world, where it's all or nothing, this book is here to introduce some much-needed nuance. If you're an ethical omnivore concerned about the environmental impact of your food choices, this book is for you. If you're a vegetarian or vegan but are considering eating meat again, like Robb was, this book is for you. If you're familiar with how cattle can be part of a regenerative food system, but still worried red meat will kill you, this book is for you. If you're open to science, then this book is *definitely* for you.

Now, some will say that we are writing this material to support positions set forth in our previous work; Robb is a Paleo diet expert and Diana has written two Paleo cookbooks. But you'll find that many of our conclusions are at odds with deeply held beliefs in the ancestral health community. Perhaps most glaring: although grass-fed meat may be superior from a sustainability perspective, current research indicates that it is only marginally different from conventionally raised meat when it comes to health and nutrients. Adherents of both veganism and the Paleo diet will take issue with much of what we have to say, and that puts us in an unenviable position as authors. It would be easier for us if our findings lined up neatly with one of these worldviews, but as you will see, the truth may not fit perfectly with any preconceived diet rules.

WHAT YOU WILL LEARN

Several years ago a PBS station in Boston was organizing a meat debate. On the anti-meat side of the aisle were to be Whole Foods CEO John Mackey and pro-vegan physician John McDougall. Robb was approached about being on the "pro-meat" side of the debate. Robb asked what the format and topics were to be. The PBS representative said it was to be a discussion on the relative health merits of a meat-inclusive diet versus a vegan diet. Robb said that was unacceptable. Discussions like this tend to involve a lot of moving the goalposts: They typically start with the health topic (although today, environment and climate change have perhaps displaced this), and as the many problems with a vegan diet become obvious, the discussion inevitably shifts to the environment. Once significant doubt emerges about the plausibility of a food system absent animals, the discussion then shifts to ethics. Once the least-harm principle and a basic understanding of food production systems is established, the topic inevitably shifts to feeding the world.

Robb insisted that both sides should make their respective cases on each of these topics and then be "cross-examined" by their debate counterparts. He would not participate in a format where his counterparts could hop from topic to topic, obscuring the topic at hand. The PBS representative thought this was a good idea and would make for a much more robust discussion. For reasons known only to them, Mackey and McDougall pulled out of the discussion once these rules of engagement were in place.

Sacred Cow will follow the same format Robb suggested for the PBS debate because a book about why we need "better meat" in our food system must address the three main criticisms against meat: nutritional, environmental, and ethical.

These important topics generate more than a few questions:

- Should we eat meat at all?
- Is there a "best" diet for humans? Or is there a spectrum of optimal human nutrition?
- Can meat be part of a sustainable food system?
- Can a sustainable food system exist *without* meat and animal contributions, both nutritionally and environmentally?
- How important are ethics in the story of human nutrition and sustainability?

There are sound cases to be made that a food system that includes grazing animals can be the best choice for our environment and our bodies, and that eating large grazing animals like cows can actually represent the path of "least harm" from an ethical standpoint. Our goal is to bring the real food and sustainability worlds together. It's time to look back toward nature to learn how to fix our future.

SACRED COW QUICK REFERENCE GUIDE

We recommend reading *Sacred Cow* from start to finish, but we also realize some of you may be itching for answers to your most burning concerns about beef. To help you tackle the book in this way, here's a list of the most common questions so you can skip to the relevant section:

1. Do vegetarians live longer than meat eaters? Page 61.

2. Will eating meat increase my chances of getting cancer? Page 56.

3. Aren't we eating way too much meat? Page 31.

4. How much protein should I eat? Page 32.

5. Is grass-fed beef healthier than typical beef? Page 73.

6. Isn't it possible for me to get all my nutrients from plants? Chapter 6 (page 85).

7. Are lab-meat and hydroponics a good way to grow food? Page 129.

8. Don't cattle emit "too much" methane? Page 134.

CHAPTER 1

MEAT AS SCAPEGOAT

It's commonplace today to blame meat for everything from cancer to global warming. We hope you can appreciate that addressing all these claims is a bit like a game of whack-a-mole. That said, in the last several years that we've both been talking about the benefits of better meat, we've been able to boil down the arguments against meat into three main subjects: nutrition, environment, and ethics. During any debate, once we've thoroughly addressed the nutritional case, the argument swiftly shifts to greenhouse gases, land use, water, sentience, intent, or least harm. Before we begin to unpack these, let's begin with our current situation: the climate crisis and our failing health, and why we believe cattle are being unfairly blamed as one of the main culprits.

We appear to be in the midst of the sixth mass extinction the earth has witnessed since life began. About 40 percent of our insect population is on the decline, and according to one study the earth may not have any insects at all by 2119.[1] Another study found that over the last hundred years, the average rate of vertebrate species loss was one hundred times the normal rate.[2] When we lose one specific plant that was the primary food for an animal, that animal dies, and the larger animals that depend on the first animal are also threatened. Across the 4.5 billion-year history of the earth, mass extinction events are certainly not unheard of; there have already been five mass extinctions in which 75 percent of the planet's living species died off. This extinction, however, is different from the others because it is largely attributable to habitat loss—which is thought to be due to intensive agriculture and agrochemical pollutants.[3]

At the same time life on the planet is suffering environmental threats, human health is also getting worse. A fairly consistent feature of the twentieth century was that, in general, each generation lived longer, "better" (albeit a highly subjective term), healthier lives than the generation that came before. A host of factors played into this, not the least of which were the germ theory of infection, antibiotics, public health, and a dramatically improved diet. Yet now, for the first time in modern history, human life span, particularly in developed nations, is declining.* Chronic degenerative diseases are rapidly increasing. And despite knowing more about nutrition than ever before, our obesity and diabetes rates continue to soar. Throughout recorded history, hunger has been humanity's main problem. But today, far more people die from eating too much rather than too little—although it's fair to say that most of these people are overfed yet undernourished (a topic we will explore more later). What's more, the real health-care costs associated with our broken food system are poised to literally cripple developed countries via a host of untenable economic scenarios. One in seven dollars spent on health care in the US goes to treating diabetes and its complications,[4] and the combined cost of health care and missed work from obesity is over $150 billion.[5]

We're rightly scared about our health and our world. But many of the proposed solutions have tunnel vision. More and more, we are being sold a notion that there is only one "good" way to eat and,

---

* There are a few small caveats and deviations from this trend, and as we will see when we consider the dietary practices of the mid-Victorian era, human health has alternated from good to poor, to good, to poor . . . all based on the relative quality of the available diet.

by extension, only one way to produce food. Christiana Figueres, the former executive secretary of the United Nations Framework Convention on Climate Change, recently declared that eating meat should be abolished. "How about restaurants in 10–15 years start treating carnivores the same way that smokers are treated? If they want to eat meat, they can do it outside the restaurant."[6] But is meat eating really as toxic as smoking cigarettes? Is a global food system really most sustainable if it focuses on a few crops, which are dependent on synthetic fertilizers and pesticides? How did we get to this point, where food sources that humans have relied on for millions of years are now considered backward and objectionable?

A BRIEF HISTORY OF HUMANS AND FOOD

Meat is strong. It's red, bloody, has a rich flavor, and throughout our history has been associated with hunting, ritual, power, vitality, sexuality, and wealth. And as we'll discuss later (chapter six), animal products are nutritionally vital to humans. Despite the nutritional benefits of meat, plant proteins are labeled as "pure" and "clean" while meat and animal products have been labeled as dirty, unhealthy, and sinful. Many people classify their diet as it relates to the level of meat intake (carnivore, omnivore, vegetarian, flexitarian, or vegan) and there are strong judgments made by some of these dietary tribes against each other.

This is *not* new. Within just the Abrahamic religions, differing food proscriptions have helped to define culture and demarcate in-groups from out-groups. But "we" are modern, civilized, and sophisticated. Surely, ancient tendencies to define good versus evil, to call for violence against another group based on food, is a feature of our past, not our future. Right? How did meat go from a necessity to something many fear or even are repulsed by?

Frédéric Leroy, a food scientist and microbiologist at the Vrije Universiteit Brussel, has written on the topic of meat and how our views of it have changed through the years. Leroy has examined how meat became a "pharmakon," a Greek word that can equally denote a remedy and a poison, as well as a "pharmakos," or scapegoat.[7] This idea has grown in lockstep with increasing concerns about our health and environment and may have roots in our collective disconnect from how food in general—and meat in particular—is produced. An alternate title for this book could have been *Scapegoat*, as meat is a singular focus of all that is wrong with the modern world, including individual health concerns, privilege, and "destroying the planet." No other food is quite as powerful or polarizing. We'll dig more into this idea in chapter fourteen, but it's critical to note that the feelings we have toward killing animals are deeply entrenched in our culture, and this has influenced dietary and environmental policy.

Humans weren't always separate from nature, or at least not as contemporary Westerners are now presenting the issue. As hunter-gatherers for most of our existence, we held very distinct worldviews. Current research suggests that at least 2.6 million years ago animal products became an important part of the hominin diet.[8] We were able to handle raw meat by using tools to cut and pound it. Even though cooking meat didn't start until about half a million years ago, the nutrients we got from raw meat and fat gave us a huge boost, allowing for the development of bigger, smarter brains and advanced vocal cords.[9] Eating meat also gave us freedom from the time-consuming process of gathering plants and chewing them. On a calorie-by-calorie basis, animal products provide far more nutrition than any plant material, and raw, unprocessed plants required far more energy and resources to digest, so animal products were highly prized. We hunted what we needed and used all parts of the animal. Meat was important to us, both physically and as part of community function.

Beginning about ten thousand years ago, in the first agricultural revolution, human societies gradually transitioned from hunting and gathering to farming, and we began to rely more heavily on crops. Because animals were valued as labor (oxen for plowing) and grains were cheaper, eating meat was more celebratory or sacrificial and symbolic. It became a food that only the wealthier classes could afford and took on a bigger sense of power. Farming meant we had more reliable food supplies to support bigger, denser populations—so small settlements of people gradually grew into cities.

Human health took a decline during this time. We started working more as we strived to produce more food than we needed. Class systems formed, with landowners on top and those who worked to produce the food below them in the hierarchy. We lived more closely to each other—allowing for cultural development, but also for the rapid spread of disease.

Much like today, technological innovations that made farming easier and more productive also brought the risk of damaging the land. The development of irrigation systems (around eight thousand years ago) and the plow (around five thousand years ago) allowed us to produce far more food, but it was at the price of soil fertility.

This greater food production led to an explosion in the human population. Over an amazingly short period in history—from 1900 to 2011—the world's population grew from 1.6 billion to 7 billion. Between the 1950s and late 1960s a series of innovations (fertilizers, pesticides, and high-yield crops) led to a huge increase in crop production, known as the Green Revolution. Changes in how we produce and distribute food have, on the whole, helped us to increase our supply of food to support the world's population (although, of course, food scarcity remains a major problem in some regions). We now live in a time of industrial agriculture. As we entered the industrial era and moved into cities, meat production and slaughter was pushed farther and farther out of sight. Religious health reformers tried to stem the tide of immoral behavior and communicable disease by promoting bland diets and avoidance of sinful foods like alcohol, sugar, and meat. They associated meat eating with "impure thoughts," including masturbation, which was considered heinous and sinful. Conversely, adopting the God-given "Garden of Eden Diet" (fruit, nuts, vegetables, and seeds) was considered a means of salvation.

As we become more globalized and access to Western foods penetrates developing countries, the entire world is now rapidly adopting a Western diet. Worldwide, traditional, healthy foods like meat and traditional fats are being abandoned in favor of ultraprocessed seed oils and highly refined wheat, corn, and soy.

Refrigeration lets us keep our food longer and transport it farther. And, notably, the invention of synthetic fertilizers has dramatically increased crop yields—though, as we will see, not without a price. And now, highly processed and refined foods are becoming more common; on supermarket shelves and in our homes, at least in the West, food products have taken the place of whole fresh foods. For the first time in our history, humans in the West are overfed and at the same time undernourished, and yet in developing countries, they are finally starting to get the nutrients like high-quality protein and iron (from meat) they need for healthy brains and bodies, allowing them to compete with Western countries in the global market.

Today, in what can be considered a "postdomestic" society, many consider the act of eating meat barbaric. It's labeled as unhealthy, unsustainable, and morally reprehensible. These attitudes stem from our lack of connection to food production and nature itself, but government guidelines that prop up industrial agriculture and further entrench biased research are also to blame.

The story of how refined foods have taken such a prominent role in our food system may not be as riveting as a spy novel, but it does involve a good amount of political maneuvering, plus the existential threat of nuclear annihilation posed by the Cold War.

LET'S TAKE A QUICK BREAK AND DEFINE SOME TERMS THAT WE'LL BE USING QUITE FREQUENTLY IN THE BOOK.

Processed food: Food that has been altered from its fresh state. For example, freezing vegetables or canning tomatoes is processing that food. Cheese, yogurt, and dried beans are all processed foods.

Ultraprocessed food: We use this term when we refer to any food made in a factory with additives like dyes, flavor enhancers, or artificial preservatives. In general, this is most of the food found in the center aisle of the grocery store. And yes, even the products in the center aisle of Whole Foods are generally ultraprocessed.

Hyperpalatable food: Foods that are so delicious (palatable) that they can stimulate us to overeat them. These are ultraprocessed foods that combine certain flavor combinations, usually carbohydrates and fat but also may include other additives that light up those reward sensors in your brain. Examples of these foods include mac and cheese, pizza, potato chips, and French fries.

Nutrient-dense food: A food's nutrient density refers to how many micronutrients (vitamins and minerals) per calorie of food. Alcohol and sugar have a lot of calories but not a lot of micronutrients, so they're calorie dense but not nutrient dense. Meat and vegetables, on the other hand, are nutrient dense.

Industrial row-crop agriculture: We also call this "chemical" or "monocrop" agriculture. When you fly over the country and look down on all those squares and circles on the ground, that's generally industrial row crops of corn, soy, and wheat. We will show in the environmental section how this agriculture system destroys soil and entire ecosystems.

Organic agriculture: Farming that doesn't use chemical pesticides and herbicides. The origins of the organic movement intended the term to mean sustainable or regenerative (see below), but today the term has largely been co-opted by large companies that still use unsustainable farming methods and simply apply "organic" approved chemicals.

Sustainable agriculture: There is no definitive definition of *sustainable*, but we will use this term interchangeably with the term *regenerative agriculture*. The idea behind the sustainability movement is that proponents want to institute a food production method that can be "sustained" throughout time.

Regenerative agriculture: This is the latest term in the cutting-edge movement of farmers who are looking to go "beyond sustainable" and actually rebuild the soil in their food production practices. Many who promote regenerative practices criticize organic and sustainable methods as not doing enough; however, many food producers who have been in the organics and sustainability movement have exactly the same intention as those in the regenerative movement. The reason we also use the term *sustainable* is because many people don't know what *regenerative* truly means, including (unfortunately) many of the proponents of regenerative agriculture. Both authors feel strongly that animals are a critical component of any regenerative food system.

Typical beef: Also called feedlot-finished beef or industrial beef, these cattle start out on ranches grazing for the first half to two-thirds of their lives, and the last four to six months are spent on a feedlot where they are given a diet that quickly increases their weight.

Grass-fed/grass-finished beef: These are generally cattle that have grazed on pasture their entire lives, although the certifications can sometimes be contested among producers and the USDA has no official certification. Because of this, some complain that typical beef producers can call their beef "grass-fed" even though they finish the cattle on grain. Each certification has its own official definition of "grass-fed." When we refer to grass-fed beef, we mean grass-finished beef.

Well-managed cattle: We will describe this in more detail in the environmental section, but when we refer to well-managed cattle, we're referring to ranchers who move their cattle frequently to new pasture, which is healthier for the animals and the land. There are various other terms for this, including rotational grazing, mob grazing, cell grazing, intensive management, adaptive multi-paddock management (AMP), and holistic management or holistic planned grazing. Each of these terms has its own definition. The basic idea is that these ranchers are not simply putting their animals out on the same patch of land for an entire season—they are moving them often, and adapting to changes as necessary.

Concentrated animal feeding operation (CAFO): These are also sometimes called "factory" or "industrial" farms and are technically defined as housing a thousand or more "animal units" for forty-five days or more. A thousand animal units is equivalent to 1,000 head of beef cattle, 700 dairy cows, 2,500 pigs, 125,000 meat chickens (broilers), or 82,000 laying hens. The majority of the meat we eat in the United States is produced from the CAFO system.

Better meat: This book makes the case for *better* meat, meaning meat from animals that are raised in a way that mimics natural systems, like well-managed cattle or eggs from chickens with access to pasture.

SNACKS FOR THE COLD WAR

For the people who lived through its horrors, World War II was a pitched battle for existence. As the war effort ramped up, just about everything you can imagine was in urgent demand: metals, including iron for tanks and brass for bullets; rubber for tires and hoses; and of course, food. (As the saying goes, "An army marches on its stomach.") In an effort to keep our military supplied and fed, as well as feed our many allies, the US government enacted a series of incentives programs called subsidies to encourage farmers to produce as much food as possible.

The gambit clearly worked. But after the war, the US government attempted to roll back the subsidies programs—a highly unpopular proposition to the farmers who were doing pretty well with these favorable price controls. Some of the subsidies were rescinded, but many remain in place to this day.

And then there was the Cold War, a game of brinkmanship that could have ended most of life on earth via thermonuclear annihilation. It proved to also be incredibly expensive for both the US and the then USSR. Abroad, the US was embroiled in the Vietnam War, while at home the prices for food and most other commodities were increasing at a painful rate.

It may seem a stretch to link the Cold War to our current obesity epidemic and billion-dollar junk food industry, but in a fascinating article in the *Guardian*, investigative reporter Jacques Peretti traced the origin of our problem to Richard Nixon's Cold War maneuvering.[10] Peretti relates how Richard Nixon, mired in controversy at home and abroad, needed the economy to improve (or at least appear to improve) and to secure a large dedicated voting bloc; to bring down the prices of food, Nixon needed America's farmers to come on board, so he appointed an academic from Indiana, Earl Butz, to create a plan.

Butz's solution? Pay farmers to produce massive grain surpluses. The glut of corn, wheat, and other subsidies brought prices down (if you ignore the allocation of tax revenue in this scheme) and earned

Nixon the loyalty of the conservative voting bloc, which was largely represented by farmers. Tricky Dick got his votes, the US citizen now had access to cheap food, and in fact there was so much food folks had to get creative about what to do with it. Peretti writes,

> By the mid-70s, there was a surplus of corn. Butz flew to Japan to look into a scientific innovation that would change everything: the mass development of high fructose corn syrup (HFCS), or glucose-fructose syrup as it's often referred to in the UK, a highly sweet, gloppy syrup, produced from surplus corn, that was also incredibly cheap. HFCS had been discovered in the 50s, but it was only in the 70s that a process had been found to harness it for mass production. HFCS was soon pumped into every conceivable food: pizzas, coleslaw, meat. It provided that "just baked" sheen on bread and cakes, made everything sweeter, and extended shelf life from days to years.

Around the same time (as we will see in chapter four) consumers were shifting away from animal products in the belief that saturated fat was a danger for their health. Peretti says, "The food industry had its eyes on the creation of a new genre of food, something they knew the public would embrace with huge enthusiasm, believing it to be better for their health: 'low fat.'" Peretti goes on to connect our new hunger for sugar, along with the burgeoning low-fat movement, to the escalation of a dietary disaster: people were getting fatter, and no one knew why. Dietary fat was being vilified, particularly fats of animal origin. The main solution then was to consume more carbs and vegetable oils. Conveniently, the government also began the subsidization of corn and other commodities that are easily transformed into hyperpalatable, shelf-stable, high-profit-margin junk food.

So connecting the Cold War to the junk food industry is not such a nutty idea after all.

All these events and policies have had remarkable unintended consequences, which we'll explore in more detail in later chapters.

WHAT'S THE SOLUTION?

Now we've seen, in brief, how humans went from the diet of our hunter-gatherer ancestors to our current highly processed diet. As we will learn in chapter four, research published throughout the last hundred years led us to believe that animal protein and fats, especially from beef, are a danger to our health.

Although humans are remarkably sophisticated, we have a predilection for simple explanations of our complex world. This desire for simplicity often makes researchers, politicians, and the public want to blame *one* thing for our woes. One day it was fats and the next it was carbohydrates that were blamed for degenerative disease in the Western world. More recently, some doctors and researchers have hung everything from cancer to diabetes on red meat. This is the latest iteration of the demonization of fat and meat. The idea has incredible legs and is once again influencing everything from health policy to agricultural practices. History may not repeat itself, but it does rhyme.

The depiction of red meat as our main dietary foe plays nicely into our current fears about a warming planet and the ethical and sustainability considerations of factory farming. This multitiered attack on red meat makes it out to be even more evil than fat or cholesterol ever could have been. (Ironically, it's fantastic for food manufacturers, as they may capitalize on our concerns for the welfare of animals to peddle their ultraprocessed, artificial products that, as we'll point out, are neither healthy, beneficial to the environment, nor cruelty-free.)

To many, it seems that eliminating or dramatically reducing our intake of meat is the solution to both our failing health and the warming planet. In January 2019 the EAT-Lancet Commission, a collective of nutrition experts aimed at defining a healthy, sustainable food system for the entire planet, released their recommendations. Although there was some wording that this "one-size-fits-all style" may not be appropriate in all areas, there seemed to be little allowance or acknowledgment of cultural food preferences or regional food reliance. They call for less than half an ounce of beef a day (about half a meatball), less than one ounce of poultry, and one quarter of an egg—yet plenty of grains, industrially produced seed oils, and eight teaspoons of sugar.[11] Their guidelines are aimed at correcting the health of all people on earth and intended to be the most sustainable way to eat. But what if they've gotten it all wrong?

What if we could help developing countries produce *better* meat, not discourage them from eating it altogether?

When we assume that limiting most or all meat is the answer, are we ignoring some basic truths about how the human metabolism and nature work?

Does the science really support the claims that animal-based proteins increase obesity rates, type 2 diabetes, and cancer?

Does it make sense to be irrigating vast fields of almonds in towns where drinking water has to arrive in plastic bottles?

Is the best solution to the future of protein one where we are growing food in labs?

Should there be less nutrient-dense food (meat) for the entire human population when we're seeing, for the first time in our history, people in the West are overfed and at the same time undernourished, and in developing countries they are finally starting to get the nutrients they need for healthy brains and bodies?

Should we be looking toward a future of chemically produced monocrops if we want to cure our health or our soil?

In a world of dwindling resources, what if we reduce our reliance on synthetic chemical–based farming and get back in touch with natural cycles? Shouldn't we strive for more biodiversity, not less?

Will Meatless Mondays solve our concerns about the industrial meat industry?

Will we solve our epidemics of obesity, type 2 diabetes, and iron deficiency anemia with less red meat?

Over the rest of this book, we're going to be asking some critical questions that few others seem to be addressing. As you may have surmised, this is a remarkably complex set of topics. We wish there was an easy, sound bite–worthy way of addressing all of this, but if we do our job you will soon understand why the nutritional, environmental, and ethical considerations of eating meat cannot be ignored. Hang with us as we look at the nutritional case for meat.

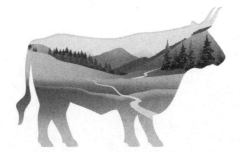

PART I

THE NUTRITIONAL CASE FOR (BETTER) MEAT

CHAPTER 2

ARE HUMANS OMNIVORES?

In his book *The Paleo Manifesto*, John Durant describes the story of Mokolo, a twenty-five-year-old gorilla living at the Cleveland Metroparks Zoo in 2005. Although Mokolo wasn't obese, he was overweight and had signs of heart disease. He also displayed odd behaviors like obsessive hair plucking. The staff realized that the best way to assess the health of a captive gorilla was to compare it to a wild gorilla. Although Mokolo was less active than a wild gorilla, he obviously didn't smoke, drink, or eat fast food. It turns out that gorillas in captivity suffer from very similar issues to those modern humans suffer from: high cholesterol, low testosterone, high blood pressure, and heart disease. In fact, heart disease is the number one killer of captive gorillas—just like it is for humans.

Realizing something needed to be done, the staff assessed Mokolo's entire environment, from the concrete floors to the light and noise levels to Mokolo's diet. He ate standard-issue "gorilla food" of fortified fiber bars, plus some plant materials like leafy vegetables and fruit. They decided one of the easiest things to change was his diet. At first, they tried increasing the fiber in the biscuits, which led to diarrhea. Next, they eliminated the fiber biscuits altogether and increased the amount of leafy plants. Because it's next to impossible to fly in native African greens, they used romaine lettuce from the local grocery store. Still, the results were astounding. Over the next few months, Mokolo lost about seventy pounds before stabilizing, and his hair plucking behavior receded.

Every animal has a biologically appropriate diet, including humans. Humans appear to thrive on a diet that is more nutrient dense than that of our great ape cousins. (Although some impassioned advocates of vegan diets will wax eloquent about the mighty gorilla, humans *cannot* process thirty to fifty pounds of vegetation per day.) In the wild, humans existed for hundreds of thousands of years on a diet that included lots of animal products, plus some honey, roots, tubers, leafy material, and fruit. But today, in "captivity," our diets have dramatically strayed from these "boring" foods in favor of highly processed food-like substances. We're also sleeping less, moving less, and under much different forms of stress than we had during hunter-gatherer times.

In our current efforts to curb the growing obesity and diabetes epidemic, many have set their sights on red meat as the culprit. Some have suggested that perhaps humans were never intended to eat meat in the first place.

You may have heard that our teeth are less like the sharp fangs of meat-eating animals and more like the flat grinding teeth of mammals that eat only plants. We don't have claws and fangs. You can even find graphics showing that human teeth are more similar to "frugivores" (animals that eat fruit, vegetables, and nuts). Are we actually biologically designed to be "peaceful" plant eaters instead of aggressive hunters and meat eaters? But, then again, can it really be the case that a food that's been part of our "wild" diet for thousands of years is responsible for our modern health woes? Let's take a look.

WHAT ARE WE PHYSICALLY DESIGNED TO EAT?

Humans have evolved an interesting mix of anatomical traits. Compared to other primates, we have larger brains, shorter large intestines, and longer small intestines. Why would that be?

In 1995 scientists Leslie Aiello and Peter Wheeler proposed an explanation in a paper published in the journal *Current Anthropology*. Their expensive-tissue hypothesis posits that in order for an animal to develop a large brain it has to prioritize fuel for the brain and use less energy in other metabolically "expensive" tissues. In humans' case, the theory goes, as our ancestors became better at procuring more nutrient-dense foods (which is arguably a feedback loop of increasing cultural complexity leading to greater ability to procure nutrient-dense food) and developed methods of preparation using tools and cooking, our digestive tract shifted, and our brains evolved. We evolved to have more real estate in the small intestine, which preferentially absorbs nutrient-dense, highly digestible foods. Relative to other primates, the fiber-fermenting portion of our digestive tract, the colon, is comparatively smaller.[1]

Varied food sources provide a more nutrient-rich diet, which is what we need. Our bodies naturally want variety, and we get bored of eating the same thing all the time. This was great when we had to go out and search for food because it kept us motivated to seek new flavors and textures. This is also why all-you-can-eat-buffets are so popular—we can try a little bit of everything![2]

It's tempting to think that the way our bodies are shaped—no claws, flat teeth—is all the evidence we need, and that we're biologically designed to eat plants. Unfortunately, what this isn't taking into account is our ability to make tools and fire. Humans can make arrows for hunting and sharpen stones and shells for scraping, pounding, and slicing meat. We don't *need* claws or massive canine teeth in order to kill and digest meat. In fact, while some other primates do eat some meat, humans consume much more.

The nutrients derived from these animal products provided to our brain is what separates humans from other primates. On the flip side, when they did consume things like grains or legumes, traditional cultures used technology to soak, sprout, and ferment them* to both reduce plant toxins and improve digestibility. Our point is that if one points to our lack of large canines as "proof" we are not designed to eat meat, is it reasonable to just ignore the technology we also needed to eat most plants?

Moving on to our anatomy, humans have distinct features that make us able to eat both plants and animals. As mentioned, our small intestines are longer than the average primate's, and our colons are smaller. This means we are not as able to break down certain plant fibers or other types of bulky plant materials (as our gorilla relatives do so well). Also, with a larger small intestine, we're adapted to eating nutrient-dense foods like meat and *cooked* starches because we are able to better absorb the nutrition from these foods. We also have different enzymes than other primates that allow us to digest dense starches and dairy. Finally, when it comes to our teeth, we have canines (for meat) and flat molars (for grinding plants). So we are equipped for chewing both plant and animal foods.[3]

We *need* nutrients that are found in both plants and animals. A study in the *American Journal of Clinical Nutrition* evaluated the diets of 229 hunter-gatherers and found that most ate somewhere from 45 to 65 percent of their calories from animal foods and the rest from plants. This practically fifty-fifty mix allows for the most variety of nutrient intake, since humans do need quite a few nutrients to thrive.[4]

By now, we hope it's clear that the argument that humans weren't "meant" to eat animals just doesn't hold water. As we saw in chapter one, humans evolved as hunter-gatherers, and when we turned to agriculture our omnivorous diet continued. Looking at

---

* And, in the case of potatoes in South America, even consume them with clay. It's speculated that the Peruvian custom of eating potatoes with a clay sauce originated in pre-Columbian times to inhibit the toxic effects of glycoalkaloids present in wild potatoes, in addition to neutralizing their bitterness.

historical records, it's very clear our ancestors ate animal products, including bone marrow, brains, muscle meat, eggs, dairy, and insects. There's no traditional human culture that excluded animal products. Although it's popular to argue that earlier societies didn't live as long as we do, it's important to note that the life expectancy figures are skewed by high infant mortality rates and the lack of modern emergency care. By and large, hunter-gatherers who survived lived quite long lives,[5] and none of these groups experienced the high rates of chronic diseases that we do now.[6] Some may dismiss this walk down our evolutionary history, but the relative good health and long life of both contemporary hunter-gatherers and our forebears is an important guidepost in human health. We have tackled this topic at length in our previous books. The takeaway is this: humans generally thrive on an omnivorous diet (both plant and animal foods).

Accepting that humans have in fact evolved to eat meat, we'll now turn to another idea: how *much* meat we should be eating.

CHAPTER 3

ARE WE EATING TOO MUCH MEAT?

When we say "too much meat," what do you think of? The visual many conjure up is that of a seventy-two-ounce T-bone steak on the American dinner plate every night. Even those who tend to agree that meat is a natural part of the human diet will often say that we're eating too much of it. (Who decides what the "appropriate" amount of meat is, the meat police?) Many people also feel that we already get too much protein and that too much protein is dangerous.

There's a lot to unpack here, so we will walk through these arguments over the next several pages. Is science driving our concept of too much, or could our perception that eating meat is an act of gluttony shape our assumptions about what is the "right" amount to eat? We'll address the science of what the right amount of meat for human consumption is soon, but before we get to it, let's talk about how much meat Americans *are* actually eating. It's less than you think, and that may be part of our problem.

SO HOW MUCH MEAT DO WE EAT?

First, let's define "meat." When folks say "meat," they're generally talking about beef. For some reason, we often separate animals into different categories (seafood, poultry, red meat). Many people will say they don't eat "meat," but they'll eat chicken or fish or eggs. Frankly, all animal proteins should be considered as such; let's call them "animal proteins" or "meat." (Categorizing fish into a "non-meat" category, as if fish aren't really "bad" or even "animals," seems illogical.)

One often hears that Americans eat 265 pounds of meat—meaning animal protein—per year. But where does that number come from?

The USDA has two sets of food consumption figures; one is "food availability" and the other is "food availability adjusted for loss." The "meat availability" figure is 265 pounds per person per year. That includes all the meat that is produced, including the chicken skin, neck, and organs, and in the case of beef, a lot of fat, organs, and other parts that don't actually make it to our refrigerators or onto our plates. We should be looking at the loss-adjusted number.

A 1,200-pound steer produces a carcass of 750 pounds, and from that carcass, about 490 pounds is retail cuts (ground beef, sirloin, and so on). The loss-adjusted numbers also factor out loss that happens between the butcher and your home, like what isn't purchased at the grocery store because of spoilage and the shrinkage that happens (water loss) when you cook meat. Another factor considered in loss is the pet food industry, which uses quite a large percentage of meat. One study found that if cats and dogs had their own country, it would rank fifth in meat consumption.[1]

In reality, we're not eating anywhere close to 265 pounds of meat per person, per year. In 2016, when adjusted for loss, Americans ate an estimated 1.8 ounces of beef per day (40 pounds per year), 1.4 ounces of pork per day (31.6 pounds per year), and 2.6 ounces of poultry per day (59.8 pounds per year).

So if we're not eating that much meat, what are we eating more of?

WE'RE NOT EATING "TOO MUCH" MEAT

Americans ate **less than 2oz of beef** per day in 2018, and global per capita beef consumption **has been flat for 50 years**. Increases in developing countries have been offset by declines in developed countries.

At the same time, **we're eating more** chicken, grains, industrially processed seed oils, and sugars.*

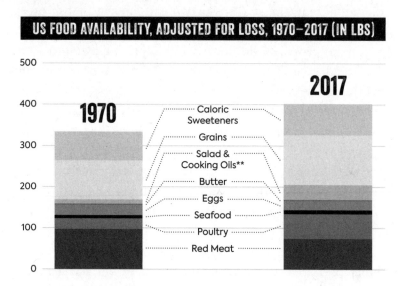

US FOOD AVAILABILITY, ADJUSTED FOR LOSS, 1970–2017 (IN LBS)

1970   2017

Caloric Sweeteners · Grains · Salad & Cooking Oils** · Butter · Eggs · Seafood · Poultry · Red Meat

* "Food Availability (Per Capita) Data System," United States Department of Agriculture, updated August 26, 2019, www.ers.usda.gov/data-products/food-availability-per-capita-data-system/food-availability-per-capita-data-system/.
** Data for Salad & Cooking Oils only available until 2010.

Since 1970 our intake of beef has actually *declined* from 2.7 ounces per person per day to 1.8 ounces per day in 2016, while our poultry intake has more than doubled.[2] We've increased our intake of caloric sweeteners, and our intake of grain products has gone up about 30 percent (and by grains, we're not talking about pearl barley; this is largely ultraprocessed foods made from wheat and corn). We've tripled our intake of ultraprocessed seed oils.

HOW MUCH PROTEIN DO WE NEED?

Now that we've covered that we're not really eating "that much" meat, how much meat do we need? You have probably heard that women need 46 grams of protein per day and men need 56 grams a day. But are these numbers correct? Where did they come from? And is there "too much" protein or meat?

According to the US Dietary Guidelines, the recommended daily allowance (RDA) is 0.8 grams of protein per kilogram of body weight. It's important to note, however, that this is a minimum requirement, not the optimal amount in order to thrive.[3] Also, just to be clear, this is grams of *protein*, not the total weight of the *food* in grams. For example, 100 grams (about 3.5oz in weight) of broccoli has 2.4 grams of protein. By contrast, 100 grams of roasted beef has 27.2 grams of protein.

Translating the RDA of 0.8 grams protein per kilogram of body weight to the public is difficult (most Americans are unfamiliar with kilograms, and many don't even know what protein is), so the folks who put together the US Dietary Guidelines decided to give actual quantities. They based the numbers on a "reference" man of 70 kilograms (154lbs) and a "reference" woman at 57 kilograms (125lbs), and calculated the numbers based on those references. So, if you go to the internet and look up, "How much protein should I eat?" the numbers you'll often find are 56 grams a day for men and 46 grams per day for women. This is also what most health professionals will tell you.

The first problem is, How many men do you know who are 154 pounds and women who are 125 pounds? The CDC says the average American man is 88.6 kilograms (195.5lbs) and the average woman is 75.6 kilograms (166.2lbs).[4] That's a big difference from the above "reference" man and woman! According to the 0.8 grams of protein per kilogram of body weight calculation, the average American man needs 71 grams of protein per day and the average American woman needs 60 grams.

The next problem? Remember, this is the *minimum* you need to avoid disease, not the "optimal" amount of protein.

The current RDA for protein intake is explained in the *Dietary Reference Intakes* by the Institute of Medicine,[5] which based their original protein recommendations on nitrogen balance studies. This gets a bit technical, so bear with us. Nitrogen balance is the difference between nitrogen intake and excreted nitrogen. It's difficult to measure, and varies greatly between individuals. It's very easy to underestimate adequate protein levels based on these studies. In fact, here is a direct quote from the report:

> In adults, it is generally presumed that the protein requirement is achieved when an individual is in zero nitrogen balance. To some extent, this assumption poses problems that may lead to underestimates of the true protein requirement.[6]

It also doesn't account for the satiating quality of protein or the nutrient density of the best protein sources. Humans don't really need "protein"; we need amino acids, and meat has the perfect balance of amino acids plus micronutrients that plants don't have. We'll dive more into that soon.

Long before the current guidelines were introduced, much higher protein recommendations were proposed. In a nutrition text from 1912, nitrogen balance studies were questioned as inaccurate measures of protein requirements, and a recommendation of at least one hundred grams of *digestible* protein (so, not just grams of total protein, but bioavailable protein—we'll get to that later) be consumed. Anything under one hundred grams a day was found to lead to ill effects.[7]

What would the "optimal" or even "adequate" amount of protein look like? There's another set of numbers we can look at called the acceptable macronutrient distribution range (AMDR). The AMDR is defined as "a range of intakes for a particular energy source that is associated with reduced risk of chronic diseases while providing adequate intakes of essential nutrients." The recommended range for protein according to the AMDR is 10 to 35 percent of caloric intake.[8] (In the 1977 guidelines the recommendation was only 10 to 14 percent).

How does this translate to our diet? The USDA estimated calorie needs per day recommends a diet of about 2,000 calories per day for average, moderately active women and about 2,600 calories per day for moderately active men. Using 10–35 percent of calories from protein, the thin reference woman at 125 pounds would need 50 to 175 grams of protein per day, and the reference man needs 65 to 228 grams of protein per day. This is a *huge* range! This makes the commonly accepted 45 grams per day for women and 54 grams per day for men below the AMDR range.

Most Americans are getting about 16 percent of their calories from protein, and a recent study showed that American adults over fifty were getting much fewer, with 46 percent not even hitting the RDA of 0.8 grams per kilogram of body weight. From the paper, "Those not meeting the protein recommendation were more likely to have intakes of other nutrients below recommended levels. Those below the protein recommendation had significantly more functional limitations across all age groups, while grip strength was significantly lower in those over 70 years old."[9]

At a conservative 20 percent of calories from protein, the average woman on a 2,000 calorie per day diet would need one hundred grams per day. This number is more than *double* the commonly assumed protein requirement of forty-five grams per day. In fact, when we're telling women to only eat forty-five grams of protein, we're recommending less than 10 percent of total calories, lower than the ADMR.* When recommending one hundred grams of protein largely from animal sources, this equals about four to six ounces of meat per meal, three times a day.

A lot of people (especially women) push back and feel like this is "too much." However, once people actually get this level of protein in their diet, they generally feel a lot better and eat less calories because they feel so full (as Diana has observed in her clinic and Robb has seen through his work, and as studies have supported). We'll get into why that is, and the nutritional benefits of meat, in chapter five.

---

* Note: The calculation for protein calories is 1g of protein for every 4 calories, so on a 2,000-calorie diet, 20 percent protein intake would equate 400 calories of protein, which equals 100g of protein.

WON'T TOO MUCH PROTEIN HURT MY BODY?

Next, let's look at that belief that eating too much protein is dangerous. You may have heard that too much protein causes too much acid in the body, or that it is useless to eat more than the minimum RDA.

The *Dietary Reference Intakes* by the Institute of Medicine actually sets no upper level for protein on the basis of chronic disease risk because high protein intake has not been found to have a detrimental effect.

You may have heard that meat is too "acidic." While it's true that urine strips can show a higher urine acid level depending on what food is consumed, the truth is that urinary pH has little to tell us about health, other than in extreme metabolic conditions, and the human body tightly controls blood pH at 7.4. Our food intake has no effect on this, and eating a more "acidic" diet from meat will not affect bone health. The research doesn't support the acid-alkaline hypothesis.[10]

What about the concerns that protein causes kidney disease and cancer? In healthy people, no danger has been found in protein intake above three grams per kilogram.[11] It's true that those with kidney disease should limit their protein intake, but there's no proof that increasing your protein intake actually *causes* kidney disease.[12] (What about all the other concerns about meat intake and chronic disease? We'll get to those in the next chapter.)

WHAT ARE THE DANGERS OF TOO LITTLE PROTEIN?

Your body needs protein, and if you don't get enough through diet, your body will start breaking down your muscles and other tissues in order to get it. This leads to muscle wasting and weakness. Immune function decreases because protein is required for antibodies. You also need protein to make enzymes and to carry oxygen to tissues, so low protein can cause lethargy. Low protein is also associated with hair loss, brittle nails, and cold hands and feet. Low protein can cause weight gain.[13] B12 deficiency, which is common in vegetarians and vegans, has been shown as an independent risk factor for coronary artery disease and serious neurological disorders in infants of vegan mothers.[14]

SO, HOW MUCH PROTEIN SHOULD YOU EAT?

In summary, it's incredibly confusing to determine how much protein to eat and the recommendations don't really seem to be based on much science, due to the inaccuracy of nitrogen balance studies and the gigantic ranges from the AMDR.

As a very reasonable starting point, it seems that 100 grams of protein on a 2,000 calorie diet is a great place to begin if you're consuming less, and many people are eating much more than 2,000 a day, so this means beef up your protein, folks. Most Americans report eating between 1,800 and 2,500 calories per day (and self-reported data is usually on the low end), so this means at 20 percent of calories, intake for many Americans should be between 90 and 125 grams of protein per day. We see great success with people upping their protein to 30 percent of total calories.

Higher levels of protein are effective for weight loss. According to the protein-leverage hypothesis, people will continue to eat food in order to satisfy their protein needs. If the food you're eating is ultraprocessed, low in protein but high in calories and carbohydrates, the brain will tell you to continue eating that food until you reach your protein minimum. Because protein is highly satiating, when we increase our protein intake, our overall caloric intake generally reduces. Protein is the most satiating of the macronutrients,[15] and intake of 15–30 percent of total calories can be quite helpful in regulating appetite by increasing leptin sensitivity and inducing weight loss and increasing blood sugar control.[16] In one meta-analysis of randomized control trials (the gold standard of nutrition research), high protein diets of 25–32 percent of calories compared to the control groups of 15–20 percent (which is still higher than the RDA), showed beneficial effects on weight loss, HbA1C levels, and blood pressure in patients with type 2 diabetes.[17]

Scientific studies show that both low fat and low carb diets can work for people,[18] but if you're looking to lose body fat and maintain muscle mass, increasing your protein and lifting some weights while being careful not to overconsume total calories (which is a lot easier to do when you're getting decent amounts of protein because you feel much more full thanks to the satiating effects of meat) is the golden ticket.[19] It also appears that chewing your food is far more satiating than drinking your calories,[20] and as we'll cover later in the book, animal proteins outweigh plant-based proteins for nutrient density. Coincidentally, increasing meat consumption also helps greatly in populations that are food insecure and need more high-quality calories, which can increase growth, behavioral outcomes, and cognitive performance in children.[21]

What does 20 percent of calories from protein look like? If you're getting this from animal foods, that looks like about twelve to sixteen ounces of meat, poultry, or seafood a day, depending on your size and specific needs. Divide that between three meals, and this is **4 to 6 ounces of animal protein per meal.** This is *not* a condiment. If you have an increased need for protein (growth, pregnancy, stress, recovery from illness, or trying to lose weight—which most of our readers likely identify with) you'll need more, depending on your size. Later, we'll talk about why animal protein is superior to plant-based proteins because it's more bioavailable, contains all the essential amino acids, and is more nutrient dense than plant-based proteins.

In this chapter we wanted to address the notion that Americans are eating too much meat. We hope you understand now that the idea of "too much" is not based on science, but more likely on a "feeling" that meat is, by nature, gluttonous and unhealthy. When you objectively look at the data, meat is a healthy food—possibly the most nutrient-dense food to humans. We aren't eating "too much," and even the RDA of protein might not be enough for our needs. Now we'll take a closer look at the findings that meat is linked to disease—and why we should take them with more than a grain of salt.

CHAPTER 4

DOES MEAT CAUSE CHRONIC DISEASE?

In the stroke of a pen we are told meat causes cancer, diabetes, heart disease. These studies have received a lot of attention in recent years and have resulted in many books, articles, and documentaries urging us to cut out meat altogether. The findings are frightening and compelling. During the writing of this book, however, a systematic review of the current research against beef published in the *Annals of Internal Medicine* surprisingly concluded that the evidence against meat is of low quality, and we in fact don't have the evidence to make public health recommendations to limit red and processed meat consumption.[1] The idea that meat might not be as bad as many want it to be is blasphemy in the plant-based world, and many in mainstream media are calling this study "controversial." Ironically, the same people who point out that the study authors have financial ties to the food industry *also* have financial ties to the food industry, books for sale that disagree with the findings, a religion-like belief in the value of observational research (we'll explain later why we disagree that nutrition policy should be set based on this type of research), or ideological biases against meat.[2] Is there strong evidence to condemn red and processed meat? Let's take a closer look.

THE CHALLENGES OF NUTRITION RESEARCH

Nutrition research is hard to do. It's usually hard to prove people were following a specific diet unless they are locked in a metabolic ward, and doing that is expensive, difficult, and short-term. Cancer, diabetes, and heart disease are not diseases that develop quickly; they take years to develop. This is why most nutrition research looks at large populations over long periods, which is called observational epidemiology. These correlational studies are not testing a specific intervention against a control group but rather simply looking at data on a specific population over time. The data could be anything from cholesterol levels to weight to cause of death. These types of studies can be either longitudinal (moving forward in time) or retrospective (looking back in time). This observational research can give us some idea into what types of connections exist between lifestyle choices and risk of a specific disease. It's a great starting point for more rigorous studies in the future. This is also where natural experiments (we talk about these later) fit into this story, as oftentimes changes occur and only later do researchers recognize an opportunity to observe what those changes may mean.

As important as observational epidemiology is, all it can really show is a *correlation*. For example, a study may find that people who eat hot dogs are more likely to die from heart attacks. But does this mean that hot dogs *cause* heart attacks? To do proper diligence, follow-up studies must be performed to tease out the different factors that contribute to this story.

Let's say people who eat hot dogs also tend to eat them with a big bun, chips, and a soda. Let's also suppose that, in general, people who don't eat hot dogs don't eat nearly as many chips or drink as much soda. In the end, can you say with certainty that it was the hot dogs themselves that caused the heart attacks? Or was it the chips, soda, bun, processed cheese sauce, or millions of other things a hot dog eater might do that a non–hot dog eater may not? Hot dog eaters, in this example, might also smoke more than the general population, not go outside as much, or tend to avoid fresh fruits and vegetables. Or perhaps the combination of hyperpalatable foods fosters significant overeating, weight gain, inflammation and dyslipidemia that is the hallmark of increasing cardiovascular disease risk? In the case of hot dog consumption and cancer, we *might* have a mechanism of causation in the form of nitrates in the hot dog. We also might have positive correlations between other things—such as the processed carb bun or overall lifestyle. It could even be that these low-cost foods are most often eaten by those who are of lower socioeconomic status, who are also more likely to be exposed to more toxins, stressful and dangerous working conditions, unsafe neighborhoods, lack of access to health care, and have less leisure time.

Do you see our point? There are so many other factors involved that could influence that connection. All these aspects, called confounding factors, must be considered. Some epidemiologists are honest that it's tough to account for all these variables. Others suggest that confounding factors, including things researchers have not yet thought to consider, can be accounted for via statistical massaging. Even when they are considered within the context of epidemiological research, it cannot be said frequently enough that the best we can find are correlations. Something that is little appreciated by researchers and the lay public alike is just how reductionistic the research of nutrition has arguably become in misguided efforts to be "scientific." The only way to truly determine a cause between two variables is to do an experimental study. In good science, we'd ideally like to change only one variable between our subjects so that we may eliminate confounding variables to test for its effects. This works well when considering the efficacy of an antibiotic or the toxicity of a given substance, but when considering the nearly infinite complexity of human diet, this approach has become something of a liability. An experimental study to connect hot dogs as a cause for heart disease, for example, would require comparing the incidence of heart attacks among research subjects confined to a baseline diet plus hot dogs for a certain period with that of another group eating the same baseline diet with *no* hot dogs, and simultaneously controlling for all other lifestyle factors like drinking, movement, stress, and sleep. Or we might feed different groups *only* hot dogs, chips, *or* soda separately, then assess their relative risks for cardiovascular disease. What we find is people given access to only one food tend to experience palate fatigue and boredom, and eat far less than if they have access to all these foods. This is a difficult topic on the best of days, and it is quite a challenge to get any information that is valuable and actionable. A remarkably persuasive way to simplify this process is to erroneously conflate causation with correlation and to steer the process toward a specific agenda. This unfortunately describes an embarrassingly large portion of nutrition research.

With observational research, it is impossible to say *x causes y* but only that there is a possible connection between the two.

Other humorous examples of the weakness of correlations can be found in Tyler Vigen's blog and book *Spurious Correlations*; one of our favorites is the graph charting the number of people who drowned by falling into a pool alongside the number of films Nicolas Cage has been in in a given year. The lines are remarkably similar. Could this be a coincidence, or does Nicolas Cage actually cause drownings in pools?

Dr. John Ioannidis, professor of medicine and of health research and policy at Stanford University School of Medicine and of statistics at Stanford University School of Humanities and Sciences, is a sharp critic of nutritional research. In his paper "Why Most Published Research Findings Are False," he explains that "research findings may often be simply accurate measures of the prevailing bias."[3]

People who eat a lot of processed meats also tend to be heavier, smoke, and engage in other activities that increase their chances of cancer. In a study called "Is Everything We Eat Associated with Cancer? A Systematic Cookbook Review" published in the *American*

Number of people who drowned by falling into a pool correlates with Films Nicolas Cage appeared in

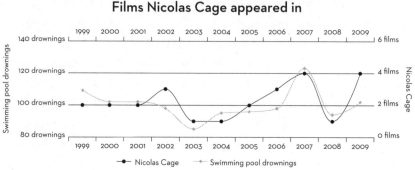

Adapted from tylervigen.com.

Journal of Clinical Nutrition, Jonathan D. Schoenfeld and John Ioannidis took fifty ingredients from random recipes out of a cookbook and searched for any evidence linking them to cancer. Of the fifty ingredients, forty had at least one study examining the cancer risk: veal, salt, pepper spice, flour, eggs, bread, pork, butter, tomatoes, lemons, duck, onions, celery, carrots, parsley, mace, sherry, olives, mushrooms, tripe, milk, cheese, coffee, bacon, sugar, lobster, potatoes, beef, lamb, mustard, nuts, wine, peas, corn, cinnamon, cayenne, oranges, tea, rum, and raisins. They found that in the majority of these studies the associations between the particular food and cancer were quite weak,[4] yet the abstract (the summary that is read by most) tended to inflate the results, making the association seem much stronger than the actual results.

Unless the food is a proved toxin, it's impossible to say *x* food **causes** *y* disease with 100 percent certainty.

Another part of nutrition research that makes determining anything with certainty really challenging is that people lie about or misrepresent their eating patterns. Most nutrition research relies on food frequency questionnaires, where subjects are asked to determine how often they eat a specific food or type of food. It has been found that **people report what they *think* they should be eating, not what they are *actually* eating.**[5] They're much less likely to "remember" the bad food they ate, and more likely to "forget" about unhealthy behaviors, like how much they drink beer and smoke cigarettes.

Let's put it this way: Do you remember how many onions you've eaten in the last three months? How about beef? (And when they ask about beef, they list foods like meatballs and tacos in addition to steak.) And how did you eat it? Were those meatballs over pasta or in a white sub smothered in cheese (with a large soda on the side)? Was the steak served over a salad, or was it in a Philly cheesesteak with a beer and side of chips? One paper found people who ate more red meat also ate more oil, potatoes, and coffee and fewer fruits and vegetables. The researchers concluded, "The association between meat consumption and a lower-quality diet may complicate studies on meat and health."[6]

How can you interpret a scientific study to determine the accuracy of the claims made? Here is a brief list of questions to ask before taking the results as a black-and-white "fact":

- What type of study was it? Observational? Experimental?
- Were there any conflicts of interest? Who paid for the study? Did a company with a vested interest in the results fund it? Were the researchers vegan or vegetarian?
- What foods were tested? How was the information about the foods eaten collected?
- How many participants? Who were the participants? Humans? Animals?
- Are the results of the study significant to overall mortality? Were they just looking at one specific compound in a food?
- If the study reports an increase in disease risk, what is the overall significance of this risk?

Given the complexity of nutrition research, if we had a scenario in which a population had a certain diet and lifestyle, and a known health and life span, then we saw a change in diet, and a change in health and life span, we might have something to think about. If the diet once again changed, and with this change a predictable outcome occurred (poor health), we have a remarkable opportunity to learn about what may constitute, if not optimum, then better human nutrition.

Unfortunately, as we will see, that's not what tends to happen; often, correlational studies are embraced as proof that a certain food leads to disease, and that tenuous connection is used as the basis for sweeping health recommendations.

DIETARY (MIS)GUIDELINES

In recent years Americans have seen recommendations shift from the "four food groups" to the "food pyramid" to the current MyPlate. On the surface, the recommendations made by academia and the government seem reasonable: eat less, particularly fat and animal products, and move more. But we have a pesky little problem—these recommendations keep failing. Failing to keep Americans fit. Failing to keep Americans healthy.

For nearly fifty years the US government told the world that a diet high in saturated fat and dietary cholesterol would increase our likelihood of everything from cancer to diabetes to heart disease. Not long ago a retraction was published saying, in effect, that there is no connection between dietary cholesterol and fat intake and the aforementioned diseases. This did not make many headlines, but it should have been a remarkable moment in history given the time, money, and effort that had been put into selling this narrative.

One day it's "high carb," the next it's "low carb." This gets pretty damn confusing, especially when we observe a variety of cultures that eat both more and less fat or carbs than Americans yet have generally better health than we do. It seems that neither researchers nor the government are looking at the continued failure of our food recommendations to try to actually make us healthier, like Mokolo's keepers did in the example in chapter two.

Hunger is an important driver and people generally eat ad libitum, which literally translates to "at one's pleasure." This works great in the "wild" when our options are some berries, a wood-grilled fish, and a roasted root, but not so great when faced with the never-ending pasta bowl at Olive Garden, a tub of ice cream, or a sleeve of Oreo cookies. We order off menus or open the refrigerator door and eat to satiety. Of course, the convenience store, the break room at work, and the pantry at home have dozens, if not hundreds, of snack options . . . The world was just created that way, right? Many of these foods have been engineered to be hyperpalatable. Some would argue they are literally addictive; for example, in recent years some researchers have gone so far as to compare sugar to cocaine.[7] The assertion that a food (or the food-like substances that comprise most of the center aisles in a grocery store) could actually be addictive is controversial, but we bet just about everybody has a favorite food that nearly makes them scream, "I wish I knew how to quit you!"

Many nutrition and medical experts counsel "moderation" and "finding balance." Although well intentioned, the advice is not only ineffective—it may even be injurious to people, as they blame themselves for "failure" instead of calling into question well-intentioned but terrible advice.

When our cars break down, we turn to a mechanic, usually with decent results. When our diets are broken (as evidenced by excessive weight or various health problems) we tend to turn to doctors and dietitians. Unlike auto mechanics, however, these folks get paid whether or not they give us good advice or produce favorable results. The standard registered dietitians, physicians, and academics who tell us to "eat whatever you want, just in moderation" are setting us up for failure, poor health, and a shorter, harder life.

When we look at moderation as a strategy for weight loss and improving health, does it work?

PREVALENCE OF OBESITY AMONG US ADULTS AGES 20–74

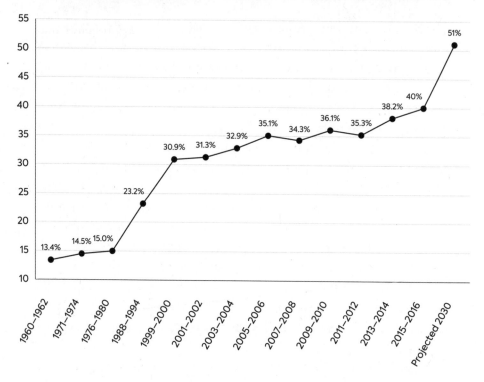

Data from *National Health and Nutrition Examination Survey, 2015-2016* and the *American Journal of Preventive Medicine.*[8]

As it turns out, a 2016 study from the University of Georgia set out to evaluate how people define moderation with food. The more someone liked a specific food, say pizza, the more pizza that person felt was a "moderate" amount. Participants tended to define "moderate" as more than what they personally ate to justify their own intake, and defended their current consumption of most foods as "appropriate." So, whether they were eating one chocolate-chip cookie daily or ten, moderate was always more than what they personally consumed.[9] Funny how we justify things, isn't it? Would you ever ask an alcoholic how much beer was a "moderate" amount? Yes, "moderation" might work for a few people, but the failure rate that occurs from this approach is monumental and unsustainable.

When compared to "everything in moderation," just about *any* nutrition intervention works better. That may sound hard to believe, but it's true: studies have found that the dietary approaches that limit options (such as vegan, Paleo, low carb) consistently work better than the academy recommendations that focus not on food quality but portion control and moderation.[10]

(There is an additional layer of irony to this story: although most of dietetics dismisses low-carb, high-protein diets as "fads," the primary complaint against this type of eating is that it "excludes whole food groups." Yet these same people and organizations routinely recommend vegetarian and vegan diets, even for children. How can one critique one nutritional strategy yet endorse another, when *both* present the same circumstance of "excluding whole food groups," and a vegan diet by default is excluding essential *nutrients*?) If a diet requires supplementation, is it a healthy diet?

Yes, portion size matters, but it appears that in the context of today's ultraprocessed food landscape, limitless food options make portion control difficult. What if the very idea of "moderating" hyperpalatable modern foods is actually going against the grain of human physiology and evolution? Whether you care to consider a low-fat vegan diet, a high-protein, low-carb diet, or something in between, the eating strategies that consistently get results have something in common: to some degree, they all limit our food options.

How did we end up in our current predicament? One need not don a tinfoil hat to realize a few large corporations make a remarkable amount of money when our gatekeepers such as dietitians, doctors, and health educators tell us to "eat everything you want, just do it in moderation."

If you think we're paranoid, consider this: in a joint initiative with the American College of Sports Medicine, Coca-Cola has invested millions of dollars into a campaign called "Exercise is Medicine" to include personal training as part of the Affordable Care Act. Now, having an insurance company reimburse you for the cost of a personal trainer may sound like a great idea, but here's the catch: Coke wants the "official" story to be that what you eat (and drink) does not matter, what matters is how much you exercise.[11] But research shows the opposite; you can't out-exercise a poor diet.[12] We see a suspiciously high rate of cardiovascular disease and other systemic inflammatory problems with elite athletes who consume prodigious amounts of refined carbohydrates.[13] Bad food will eventually catch up with us, be that in an expanding waistline or a trip to the cardiac care unit.

How our governmental policies have become so divorced from what the research *really* shows is a topic worth exploring.

KEYS TO THE KINGDOM

One of the biggest criticisms against red meat is that it is high in saturated fat, and we all know that saturated fat will clog your arteries and give you a heart attack, right? Well, it turns out, no. Eating fat doesn't equate to more fat in the blood.

Some experts have been making gains in reversing the widespread bias against fat. However, decades of fear of fat and cholesterol aren't so easily erased. It all started with a researcher named Ancel Keys.

Keys was a remarkable individual with an eclectic background ranging from chemistry to zoology and economics. He managed to dramatically alter the course of US and global food policy. His interests led him to studying human nutrition and disease using the tool of epidemiology—the study of disease across populations. Keys and other researchers observed that Americans were a bit heavier and suffered from cardiovascular disease more than many other Westernized countries, so he spearheaded a study in the early 1950s called the Seven Countries Study, which would become one of the most influential scientific studies in the history of nutrition. The basic purpose of the study was to look at the amounts of saturated fat, particularly from animal sources, consumed in various countries relative to the rates of death from cardiovascular disease.

Keys's data pointed to a nearly perfect correlation between higher fat intake and deaths from cardiovascular disease; Japan, which had the lowest percentage, had the lowest incidence of heart disease, while Canada and the United States, with the highest percentage of calories from fat, had the highest.

Keys's findings received a boost of sorts when health data from post–World War II Europe was analyzed. Certain countries saw a marked decrease in cardiovascular disease both during and immediately after the conflict. The war had dramatically altered trade, and there were shortages of just about every commodity you can think of. Folks had to rely on homegrown produce to meet their basic needs, and consequently ate less fat, sugar, and calories overall. Despite the fact that several important dietary factors had changed, supporters of the "dietary fat = disease" theory ascribed the improved health solely to the reduced fat intake.

Keys's findings might have remained a possibly interesting footnote in medical research history, but the formation of a governmental committee, initially tasked with addressing the problem of malnutrition in the US, provided the catalyst to launch government and business into the "macronutrient wars." The US government accepted Keys's work and began recommending low-fat diets to everyone. (The recommendation to avoid saturated fat is *still* a part of American dietary guidelines.)[14] However, many people in the research community at the time were highly critical of Keys. His work was rich in correlation yet anemic in causation. Although some of Keys's research suggested a link between fat intake, blood cholesterol levels, and cardiovascular disease (CVD), there was perplexing data showing examples of higher fat intakes and lower rates of CVD, and also lower fat intakes and higher rates of CVD (all relative to the US). Despite these inconsistencies, Keys was tenacious in promoting his hypothesis and developed a reputation for publicly attacking dissenting voices in a way that would have likely made him successful in a modern presidential campaign. We think it's fair to say he did not consider other factors such as sugar and refined carbohydrate intake.

Another interesting but ultimately misleading study contributed to our misunderstanding of what causes heart disease: earlier in the twentieth century, pathologist Nikolai Anichkov performed a study in which rabbits were fed either a low- (none) or high-cholesterol diet. The rabbits who ate large amounts of cholesterol developed damage and blockage to the arteries at high rates. This was a remarkable finding in that it linked cholesterol to cardiovascular disease, but again, the story is much more complex than first meets the eye. (This is a good place to circle back to Mokolo and the idea of the "ancestral diet" of any organism.) Some critters eat plants, others eat animals, and some eat both. The digestive and metabolic physiology of an herbivore is dramatically different from that of a carnivore or omnivore. Dietary cholesterol, a product found exclusively in animals, would of course create serious problems for rabbits—they are not wired to eat animal products.

Cholesterol is one of the most contentious topics in all of medicine. One camp clamors that we should endeavor, by any means necessary, to drive cholesterol levels as low as possible to avoid disease. On the other side are folks who claim there is *no* relationship between cholesterol and the development of atherosclerosis and cardiovascular disease. As with most topics, the devil is in the details. We will look at the specifics later, but the takeaway is that the rabbit cholesterol studies were important in suggesting a potential mechanism for cardiovascular disease. But these studies were also taken out of context; as we'll see, they played into a larger story picked up by researchers and politicians who were influenced by work like that of Ancel Keys. (Incidentally, Keys was clear in stating that dietary cholesterol was not a factor in cardiovascular disease, but many high-fat foods are also rich in cholesterol. In the process of demonizing dietary fat, cholesterol was dragged along for the ride.)

Ancel Keys, via his influence on a key governmental commission, is clearly an important figure in the formation of modern dietary policies. In 2016 an interesting paper emerged that looked at research led by Dr. Ivan Frantz Jr., one of Keys's close associates.[15] The original work was part of the Minnesota Coronary Experiment, which ran from 1968 to 1973. This was one of the largest and best-conducted controlled studies of its kind. It would literally be impossible to do a study like this today, owing to both costs and ethical considerations. Over nine thousand hospitalized mental patients were fed either a diet rich in saturated fat or a diet in which the saturated fat was replaced with polyunsaturated fats from vegetable oils. The patients fed vegetable oils showed a decrease in cholesterol levels but, interestingly, no decrease in mortality. In fact, the opposite was seen; the patients fed vegetable oils were more likely to die during the study period than those fed saturated fat, who coincidentally had higher cholesterol levels. This original material was not published until 1989, and, oddly, that publication claimed there was no difference between the two groups.[16] Recent analysis of the raw data has left many in the research community scratching their heads as to why this information took so long to be released, and upon release did not accurately reflect what the data suggested.[17]

What should we make of this? One might suspect that the information was suppressed to forward Keys's low-fat position, but we really do not know why this situation played out as it did. What is clear is that a large, well-controlled study, influenced by Keys's own work, casts serious doubt on the notion that saturated fat and elevated cholesterol are the drivers of cardiovascular disease.

McGOVERN COMMISSION— OR SCIENCE BY COMMITTEE

Exactly what influence the government should play in our lives is a hot topic—one that, if booze and heated political debates are allowed to mix sufficiently, could turn any polite family gathering into a crime scene. Wherever you may be on the political spectrum, there is no doubt that the government *does* influence our lives.

The Select Committee on Nutrition and Human Needs, headed by Senator George McGovern, was founded in 1968 and was tasked with addressing the problem of undernutrition in the US. The committee achieved a laudable degree of success in this regard, but as is often the case with governmental agencies, when the initial charter of the committee neared completion, the committee was not disbanded. Instead, it was repurposed and given the new directive to formulate dietary guidelines to reduce the rates of disease afflicting Americans, including heart disease. The people tasked with this process were not scientists but rather lawyers and clerks, many of whom were passionate about the idea of vegetarian and low-fat diets.

After hearings and consultations with a vegetarian-leaning nutritionist from Harvard University, initial guidelines were released with the recommendation to increase carbohydrates and decrease fat, particularly saturated fat. The recommendations were not warmly received and were broadly criticized within the scientific community. Interestingly, those scientists who argued there was scant evidence to support the notion that health would be improved by the reduction of fat, meat, and eggs were dismissed as being shills for the meat and dairy industries.[18] Money certainly influences policy; nobody can argue against that. But when the government picks "winners" by casting its lot in with a specific dietary approach, and that approach is later propped up by government subsidies, we are not talking about equal influence or outcomes.

Despite the pushback from the scientific community, the notion that reducing fat intake, particularly from animal sources, would improve health was sexy. It was the tail end of the Vietnam War, the "establishment" was the enemy, and many of the staples of American culinary experience such as steak, eggs, and butter were falling out of favor owing to the rise of "enlightened" cuisines that focused more on beans and whole grains.

The burgeoning vegetarian movement, coupled with questionable nutrition research and guidelines, resulted in a shift in governmental food recommendations toward more carbohydrate and less fat intake. When scientists asked for time to collect more data to support these changes in dietary recommendations, Senator McGovern quipped, "We Senators don't have the luxury that a research scientist does of waiting until every last shred of evidence is in."[19]

Between Keys's research and the McGovern commission's rush to deliver results, the stage was set: dietary fat, once a staple, would soon be viewed as a sin.

Given our position thus far, you may think we are Luddites who eschew all modern advances. Far from it. Modern medicine is a miracle. If you have a bullet wound, get hit by a bus, or contract a wacky tropical virus, you have a better chance of survival today than ever before in history. But the medical establishment has produced a few recommendations that haven't aged well. Fifty years ago your doctor might have prescribed a "healthy" cigarette brand.[20] Fifty years from now we bet it will be just as absurd that the medical establishment now puts its hallowed seal of approval on nearly anything, provided it's low fat (and isn't red meat).

All that said, we're going to present a perspective that will ruffle some feathers in the low-carb camp: had the dietary recommendations born of Ancel Keys's work (eat less fat and more carbs) and bolstered by the McGovern commission been implemented in a whole food fashion, it may not have really been that big of a deal. The recent DIETFITS randomized clinical trial placed participants on either a *whole food–based* low-fat or low-carb diet and tracked their progress for thirteen months. This is a well-designed study that not only provided ongoing education, support, and monitoring to help ensure adherence but also looked for genetic markers that might suggest one diet or the other would be a better fit for any given individual. **Protein intake was equal and adequate in both groups!** We'll come back to this point several times throughout the rest of this chapter, as adequate protein intake, without too much in the way of processed foods, may be the recipe for dietary success.

The results? In general, both groups lost significant amounts of weight and improved their health, though some people within both groups actually fared worse.[21]

What this research (and more than twenty years of personal experience) suggests is different people do better or worse on different eating programs. When working with nutrition clients, both of us use low-fat and low-carb approaches, but in a "real food" context. But the sad fact is that the well-intentioned message to eat less fat was myopic given our ultraprocessed food environment and variability within human populations. Worse, this all-or-nothing message of "reduce fat intake at all costs" was all too easily co-opted by the nascent junk food industry and was shocked into life via government stimulus to win votes and assuage concerns about national food security during the Cold War. The net effect on the medical community and most of society was "so long as it's low fat, it's OK."

So, clearly, there are a lot of issues with nutritional research and the recommendations that come out of it. Over the next several pages we'll take a look at some of what you may have heard about meat and chronic disease—and, we hope, put your fears to rest.

DOES MEAT CAUSE CANCER?

The research around meat and cancer is a fascinating exploration of how even the best of intentions may, if not make things worse, make them quite oblique. The idea that meat may play a role in cancer has been a feature of both research and mysticism for over a hundred years. The source most often cited is the World Health Organization (WHO), which leans heavily on the work of the International Agency for Research on Cancer (IARC), which categorizes different substances or "agents" into the following groups:

Group 1	Carcinogenic to humans	120 agents
Group 2A	Probably carcinogenic to humans	81
Group 2B	Possibly carcinogenic to humans	299
Group 3	Not classifiable as to its carcinogenicity to humans	502
Group 4	Probably not carcinogenic to humans	1

The most often-cited material places meat, particularly processed meats, among the group 1 carcinogens, along with a host of substances including tobacco, various viral infections, alcohol, and plutonium. News reports and documentary films such as *What the Health* have concluded that meat is "as bad" as smoking or exposure to radiation.

But let's not be so hasty. In an interview for Cancer Research UK, Professor Phillips explains the IARC process: "IARC does 'hazard identification', not 'risk assessment'. . . That sounds quite technical, but what it means is that IARC isn't in the business of telling us how potent something is in causing cancer—only whether it does so or not." To make an analogy, think of banana peels. They definitely can cause accidents, explains Phillips, but in practice this doesn't happen very often (unless you work on a banana farm). And the sort of harm you can come to from slipping on a banana peel isn't generally as severe as, say, being in a car accident. But under a hazard identification system like IARC's, banana peels and cars would come under the same category—they both definitely do cause accidents.

So let's look at what IARC is actually saying about meat.

Processed meat—meaning bacon, ham, sausages and cured meats, canned meat, and meat-based sauces—is classified as group 1, "carcinogenic to humans." Also in the class 1 category, we can find "air," wine, and sitting near a sunny window. The research seems to suggest that with every daily fifty-gram increase in processed meats, there is an 18 percent increase in the risk of colorectal cancer (this is the case we made previously about relative versus absolute risk). An 18 percent increase sounds scary, right? But does that mean we need to stop eating bacon?

One slice of bacon is approximately eight grams. So, if an individual ate five strips of bacon every single day, that person's risk would go up 18 percent. Now, let's also look at what an 18 percent increase in cancer risk really means. The risk of getting cancer is 1,500 to 3,000 percent (or fifty to thirty times) higher for smokers as opposed to nonsmokers. An 18 percent increase in cancer from eating processed meat isn't even twice the risk. In the US the average rate of colon cancer is 5 percent. An 18 percent increase in this risk would move you to almost 6 percent, if you ate five slices of bacon every single day. Now, if eating five slices of bacon daily doubled your chance of contracting colon cancer, then that could be a cause for concern, but the risk is only slightly elevated (and based entirely on observational studies, which we explained previously are built from food frequency surveys—the actual risk is incredibly debatable given the potential error of these types of studies). Yet with a bit of statistical massaging, the difference between 5 percent and 6 percent (20 percent in this case, which is called the "relative risk") is what is reported and what snags the pithy news headlines. To classify processed meats and cigarettes in the same category is clearly misleading. Additionally, smoking causes more different types of cancer, including lung, mouth, throat, esophagus, liver, bladder, kidney, cervix, stomach, bone marrow, and blood.

Fresh red meat was classified as group 2, or "probably" cancer causing. By the way, so is any food that's grilled. Yet there is no strong evidence at all that fresh red meat causes cancer. None. Interestingly, a group of researchers analyzed the research that the IARC used to link red meat and processed meat to cancer. It turns out, the vast majority of the studies (about 80 percent) were in Western populations. Of the 15 percent of the studies on red or processed meat and cancer that were conducted in Asian countries, most of them showed no link between fresh or processed meat and cancer. If red meat and processed meat causes cancer, wouldn't it also cause cancer in Asians? The researchers stated, "The incidence of colorectal cancer may be related to causative factors other than meat consumption, such as ethnicity, dietary habits, alcohol consumption, smoking, stress, exercise, medical check-up frequency, or environmental pollution."[22] If there was a mechanism for meat to cause cancer, we would expect to see some evidence of a mechanism in randomized controlled trials, but this is just not the case.

DOES MEAT CAUSE HEART DISEASE?

The claims that meat causes heart disease come largely from the fear that saturated fat increases cholesterol, and that high cholesterol causes heart disease. Earlier in this chapter, we discussed how Ancel Keys incorrectly implicated dietary saturated fat as the cause of heart disease. A very large meta-analysis and systematic review of both observational and randomized controlled trials involving over six hundred thousand participants concluded that "current evidence does not clearly support cardiovascular guidelines that encourage high consumption of polyunsaturated fatty acids and low consumption of total saturated fats."[23] Again, the studies that link dietary saturated fat and cholesterol to heart disease are based on epidemiology, which can reveal associations but not causes. Dietary cholesterol has been vindicated and is no longer "a nutrient of concern" by the Academy of Nutrition and Dietetics. Once gospel, the diet-heart hypothesis has been proven wrong in many books and papers. There is no connection between dietary cholesterol and saturated fat intake and heart disease.

Still not convinced? If eating meat caused heart disease, then you'd bet that the Tsimané, the Bolivian population found to have the lowest rate of heart disease in the world, would likely have a completely meat-free diet. However, approximately 14 percent of their diet comes from seafood and game they hunt. Of course, there are many other factors to their diet and hunter-gatherer lifestyle that could be contributing to their good health, but they also tend to have a high parasite load, which leads to inflammation. A study published in the *Lancet* reported that their arteries at age eighty look like a typical Westerner's at age fifty.[24] If eating meat alone was the cause of cardiovascular disease, we'd see it in this population, but we don't.

DOES MEAT CAUSE OBESITY?

Does meat make people obese, or do people who are obese tend to eat more meat? Again, observational studies simply can't tell us. You might be thinking that you know of folks who have eliminated meat and have lost weight. While this can be true, there are two factors at play here.

The first is that when people adopt a vegan or vegetarian diet, they often also eliminate the foods that we know cause obesity—processed foods. By simply cutting out nutrient-poor, ultraprocessed foods that stimulate us to overeat, people will naturally lose weight. Second, when people reduce their overall caloric intake, they will lose weight. But weight loss is not the same as fat loss. Both low-carb and low-fat diets lead to weight loss because they usually also involve restricting calories, but what is important to note is that high-protein diets that are either lower in carbs or low in fat lead to more *fat* loss. A review published in the *Journal of the American College of Nutrition* found that the benefits of a high-protein diet were found *even when people continued to eat the same amount of calories*. Based on their findings, the authors recommended a daily intake of 1.5 to 2 grams per kilogram of body weight of high-quality protein (from animal sources).[25]

How does a higher-protein diet (at least double the RDA of 0.8 grams per kilogram of body weight) work? The first way is through simply feeling fuller. Protein is the most satiating macronutrient largely because of its effect on appetite-regulating hormones. Although caloric restriction works in lab settings, out in the real world, people generally eat to satiety, so if you feel fuller, you're less likely to overeat. When combined with weightlifting, protein increases muscle mass, so as you lose fat you gain muscle. Other diets like caloric restriction generally cause weight loss but the goal should be fat loss, not merely "weight." And, high protein diets help us to burn more fat because of something called the "thermic effect of food" (basically, that means how much energy it takes to digest the food you ate). Protein has a high thermic effect on food because it takes more energy to break it down. Interestingly, high-protein diets tend to negate having to count calories. People who followed a high-protein diet and either cut their calorie intake or kept it the same have shown to improve body composition—but people who ate *more* calories still did not seem to see increased fat mass when those extra calories came from protein. Simply put: increase protein, keeping calories the same, work out, and you will likely lose weight.[26]

Far from causing obesity, eating a higher-protein diet may be the key to helping people *regulate* their weight—a widespread problem we cannot deny. It can be easy to lose weight when you reduce calories, but if you're hungry all the time, your hunger will eventually get the better of you. Yes, plants are lower in calories, but eating more plants does not provide increased satiation. Animal protein is also far more absorbable than plant protein. If you want to meet your protein needs in plant foods alone, you will need to consume more calories (we'll get back to this idea in chapter six).

DO VEGETARIANS LIVE LONGER THAN MEAT EATERS?

You may have seen headlines that vegetarians live longer than nonvegetarians; studies of Seventh-Day Adventists found that they live six to nine years longer than the general population. An "average" American may have a shorter life span than an American *vegetarian*. But that doesn't mean vegetarians live longer because of their diet. Remember when we discussed confounding factors in research? Vegetarians are also much less likely to smoke or drink, and much *more* likely to exercise. They also tend to eat less processed foods and sugar. So, saying that meat is the *only* factor causing disease is flawed logic.

In fact, a study that looked at people who shopped at health food stores (a change that would seem to account for some of those healthier lifestyle factors) found no difference in mortality between vegetarians and omnivores.[27] And when adjusting for confounding factors, a very large recent study found "no significant difference in all-cause mortality for vegetarians versus non-vegetarians."[28]

What about those Seventh-Day Adventists? When compared to the typical American omnivore, these studies show that the Seventh-Day Adventists are less likely to have cancer or heart disease or to die from any cause. But they're not factoring in the fact that this population doesn't drink or smoke, has strong community, and lives a very healthy lifestyle overall.

If only there was a similar group that ate meat . . . Oh, wait! It turns out that Mormons practice very similar lifestyle habits to the Seventh-Day Adventists. Three studies looking at the longevity of Mormons all showed that this group has significantly better health and longer life spans than typical Americans.[29]

BUT WHAT ABOUT . . . ?

But what about mTor, TMAO, Neu5Gc, and the like? (If you don't know what those are, don't fret.) You may have heard of studies linking certain lesser-known compounds found in animal products to poor health.[30] Again, when we take a critical look at these studies, we find that they are generally not conducted on humans, and they look at isolated compounds (not whole foods like steak). We'd also expect to see very strong evidence that those reducing animal products led to longer-lived, healthier people. But that's not happening. In fact, some research suggests TMAO is beneficial (if you're wondering, that's trimethylamine N-oxide, a compound that increases in the blood after we eat foods, like red meat, that contain carnitine).[31]

Among all the components in meat that have been vilified, perhaps the only one that deserves closer attention is advanced glycation end products (AGEs). There is concern that certain types of cooking result in high levels of them, and that dietary advanced glycation end products (dAGEs) are known to contribute to increased oxidant stress and inflammation.[32] The effect of cooking that's implicated here is also referred to as the browning or Maillard reaction; it is a normal part of cooking but is thought to be problematic in large amounts. Lower-temperature cooking, moist heat, and the use of acids like lemon and vinegar all seem to reduce the formation of AGEs.

In the interest of brevity, we will devote more time on Sacredcow.info to debunking more of these antimeat health claims (that could take up the entire book!). Hopefully, though, you get the point that relying on food frequency questionnaires, pulling out one isolated aspect of the diet, and assigning blame to a particular food—especially one that has been part of the human diet for thousands of years—should be met with the highest level of skepticism.

THE MID-VICTORIAN DIET

We've spent this chapter analyzing some of the high-profile research that has been used to justify criticisms of meat. But we'd like to end it with a look at a study you may have never heard of. Quietly published in the *International Journal of Research and Public Health*, the paper "How the Mid-Victorians Lived, Ate and Died" paints a remarkable story of a group of people that underwent one of the most remarkable natural experiments in history 150 years ago.

The researchers write,

During these 30 years [between 1850 and 1880] a generation grew up with probably the best standards of health ever enjoyed by a modern state . . . Britain and its world-dominating empire were supported by a workforce, an army and a navy comprised of individuals who were healthier, fitter and stronger than we are today. They were almost entirely free of the degenerative diseases which maim and kill so many of us, and although it is commonly stated that this is because they all died young, the reverse is true; public records reveal that they lived as long—or longer—than we do in the 21st century.

Now, during this time, that population lived in unhealthy, increasingly urbanized situations, before the public health movement came about, and during an era that is remembered for its dirty cities and high disease. Still, the paper's authors argue, mid-Victorians enjoyed a standard of health comparable to ours today—all thanks to their diet. (Often, the notion that there have been populations with better health than modern people's is dismissed—and wrongly.)

So just what were they eating during this period of remarkable health? The hallmark of the mid-Victorian diet is an abundance of whole, largely unprocessed foods, produced in a manner that goes far beyond our modern standards of "organic" and grass fed. Onions were plentiful and inexpensive and generally available year-round, as were cabbage, Jerusalem artichokes, watercress, carrots, and turnips. They also ate apples, which store well through the winter, plus dried fruit, and in the summer they enjoyed gooseberries, plums, and other seasonal but more perishable fruit. They ate dried legumes and nuts. In addition, fresh and pickled fish and seafood were plentiful. All meat was "free range," and pork was the most common meat. They prepared meat on the bone, lots of stews, and ate the joints and organ meats. It was considered a poverty diet to eat limited meat. Many families kept chickens in their backyards for eggs, and hard cheeses were frequently consumed. What's more, there was a strong temperance movement that resulted in approximately a third of homes abstaining totally from alcohol. Beer was frequently consumed, but it's estimated that the alcohol content was probably only 1 or 2 percent in the home and about 2 to 3 percent at pubs, which is much lower than today's average of 5 percent.

In contrast to today's ultraprocessed diet leading to food that is calorie dense yet low in vitamins and minerals in the West, this diet is what we call "nutrient dense," meaning each calorie consumed has a high amount of micronutrients (vitamins and minerals).

The case of the mid-Victorians is what in science is called a natural experiment. When we consider the differences between experimental and observational studies depicted below, although natural experiments are technically observational, they often contain elements that are remarkably similar to the gold standard of biomedical research, the randomized controlled trial (RCT).

Clearly, we are not yet at a point where we can, at will, develop alternate dimensions to run experiments like this so we can say definitively that their good diet *caused* their good health! Still, natural experiments can tell us a lot. The main difference in the mid-Victorian diet initially was an *increase* in meat, seafood, fruits, and vegetables. Before 1850 the population had eaten a diet higher in grains. Health and longevity improved markedly alongside this improvement in dietary quality. Then, after 1880 dietary trends shifted again, becoming higher in refined foods, including significant increases in sugar, flour, and canned meats. This happened in conjunction with a reduction in vegetables, fruits, fresh meat, and seafood—and health deteriorated:

> Unfortunately, negative changes that would undermine these nutritional gains were already taking shape. Thanks to her dominant global position, and developments in shipping technology, Britain had created a global market drawing in the products of colonial and US agriculture, to provide ever-cheaper food for the growing urban masses. From 1875 on and especially after 1885, rising imports of cheap food basics were increasingly affecting the food chain at home.

Health conditions deteriorated so much that people got shorter—the infantry even had to lower its minimum height requirements for recruits.

One of the key indicators of both individual and societal health and readiness is average height. (Well-child checkups include this basic but critical piece of information.) The mid-Victorians saw a loss of half a foot in average height in approximately one generation. Human height is largely controlled by genetic factors but is incredibly susceptible to stunting when an individual or population is undernourished. Skeptics may perform a collective eye roll when talking about the significance of height and human health, but it is one of the most reliable indicators of thriving or surviving, of robust health or underlying disease. To put it simply: if a population is, on average, losing height over progressive generations, we can confidently say those shorter generations are, on average, less healthy. A recent article in the *Economist* noted that as populations increase their meat intake, not only does average height increase but so does their quality of life and longevity:

> Many African children are stunted (notably small for their age) partly because they do not get enough micronutrients such as Vitamin A. Iron deficiency is startlingly common. In Senegal a health survey in 2017 found that 42% of young children and 14% of women are moderately or severely anemic. Poor nutrition stunts brains as well as bodies.
>
> Animal products are excellent sources of essential vitamins and minerals. Studies in several developing countries have shown that giving milk to schoolchildren makes them taller. Recent research in rural western Kenya found that children who regularly ate eggs grew 5% faster than children who did not; cow's milk had a smaller effect.[33]

In America, for the first time in nearly a hundred years, both height and average life span are no longer increasing. Robb ran into this phenomenon recently when his youngest daughter attended her well-child checkup as a four-year-old. Both she and her older sister were exactly the same height and within a half a pound of weight at age four. The pediatrician commented that his youngest was in the ninety-eighth percentile of height. He asked him where his older daughter ranked. Despite the fact that both girls had been the same height at the same age, Robb's older daughter was in the ninety-sixth percentile for her age group. This was not a huge difference, but he asked the doctor about the discrepancy: same height, different percentiles? After some digging, the doctor reported, "Kids are getting shorter." It would appear that in the two-and-a-half-year age gap between his first and second daughters, the average height of children had decreased sufficiently to pop Robb's youngest into a percentile two points higher.

Some might dismiss this anecdote with a wave of the hand, but a recent study published in *eLife* looked at a hundred years' worth of human height trends and found that Americans' height has plateaued while much of the rest of the world has continued to grow.[34] This slowed growth is occurring in tandem with poorer health, higher medical costs, and a host of associated problems. As our diets become increasingly more industrialized, we're losing our nutrients and our health. Could it be worth considering—when we look at the low chronic disease rates of some traditional cultures, and the improved health of the mid-Victorians—that meat could be a part of the answer to the problems of the standard American diet?

CHAPTER 5

IS MEAT A HEALTHY FOOD?

Now that we've shown you that meat will not kill you, let's walk through some of the nutrients that animal products provide in addition to protein, which we already addressed. First, we'll address the nutrients available in meat overall, which are difficult to get from plants. Then we'll go into specific types of animal products like organ meat and seafood, as each animal species provides a unique set of micronutrients.

B VITAMINS

Contrary to what some people assume, plant foods do not contain vitamin B12. There are trace amounts of B12 analogs in foods like algae, but these are not as effective as real B12 in the body, and actually increase your need for real B12.[1] A deficiency in this vitamin can cause nerve damage, mental illness, neurological problems, and infertility; we'll look at this again in chapter six. Vegans must take a vitamin B12 supplement because it is simply not found in plant foods.

Animals are also an incredible source of several other B vitamins, including thiamin, riboflavin, pantothenic acid, B6, niacin, and folate. Each of these plays a role in energy metabolism (meaning how we use calories for energy), preventing birth defects, and a variety of other functions. Some of the best sources of B vitamins include clams, oysters, and tuna.

VITAMIN D

Vitamin D helps us to absorb calcium, so it's crucial for our bone health. Our skin makes vitamin D when exposed to sunlight, so the fact that many of us spend so much time indoors has made vitamin D deficiency incredibly common. Vitamin D comes in two forms, D2 and D3, the latter being the preferred form.[2] The best food sources of vitamin D3 are cod liver oil and fatty fish, though beef liver and eggs also contain some vitamin D. Cereals, mushrooms, and some juices are fortified with vitamin D2, which is more difficult for the body to utilize.[3]

IRON

Meat contains heme iron, the most absorbable type of iron. One study showed that when iron was fortified to teens, *only* the heme-iron fortification raised iron levels.[4] Iron deficiency anemia is the most common mineral deficiency in the US, affecting more than 25 percent of the population and almost half of all preschool children; we'll learn more about why this is a problem in chapter six. Since the prevalence of iron deficiency is so high, and given heme iron is best absorbed, those susceptible to iron deficiency should consume more liver and red meat, not less. Iron is particularly important for pregnant women, infants, and children. Clams, oysters, and liver are also great sources of iron.

IS HEME IRON BAD FOR YOU?

Some claim heme iron is associated with inflammation, cancer, and diabetes. However, when we look at all the research on this subject, it appears that there are only *associations* between those who eat meat (and therefore, consume heme iron) and disease.

Iron overload can be a serious issue for some, and there is a rare mutation to a gene called *HFE* that causes "hereditary hemochromatosis," which is thought to affect 1 in 227 people of European decent.[5] In this small percentage of the population, red meat should be avoided, but in healthy people and in those who are iron deficient, red meat is the best source of iron.

OTHER MINERALS

Meat is a great source of highly bioavailable minerals, including zinc, magnesium, copper, cobalt, phosphorus, nickel, selenium, and chromium. Plants actually can block the absorption of minerals, making meat the better way to get these in your diet. Zinc, in particular, is a common deficiency in those avoiding animal products, and zinc in animals is highly absorbable.

ANIMAL FATS

Fat from animals has been one of the most maligned foods over the last few decades. There is a constant push from the "nutrition experts" to stay away from animal fat, particularly saturated fat, as much as possible. But as we described in the last chapter, there is no evidence to support this recommendation. Long-chain fatty acids like EPA and DHA are also best found from animal products, particularly in seafood. Algae supplements can provide DHA, but there are no plant-based real food forms of this critical nutrient.

WHY EAT RED MEAT?

Although the book is primarily focused on cattle and beef, there are many other ruminant animals that are great for the environment (as we'll explain in the next chapter) and are quite nutrient dense. Chicken livers, salmon, and oysters are among some of the most nutrient-rich animal foods available, providing large amounts of B12, iron, zinc, and DHA, which are commonly deficient in a diet excluding meat.

In a 6oz serving of . . .	Vitamin B12 (micrograms)	Iron (milligrams)	Zinc (milligrams)	DHA (grams)
Beef sirloin	1.67	2.57	6.02	0
Pork chop	0.94	1.12	4.35	0.003
Chicken breast	0.58	1.26	1.36	0.034
Duck breast	0.42	**4.08**	2.31	0
Chicken liver	**28.19**	**15.28**	**4.54**	0
Salmon	**5.41**	1.36	1.09	**1.895**
Shrimp	1.89	0.36	1.86	0.119
Oysters	**14.88**	**7.84**	**66.81**	0.231

That said, beef, bison, lamb, goat, and other red meats are particularly nutrient dense and beat out poultry for most nutrients, especially for B12, iron, and zinc. Also, the fatty acid profile of beef is far better than that of poultry and pork, which are higher in omega-6 fats.

POULTRY

A four-ounce serving of chicken contains all the B vitamins, similar to red meat. Thiamin, riboflavin, niacin, pantothenic acid, B6,

N12, folate, biotin, and choline all have important functions in the body, from energy metabolism to maintaining the health of the nervous system. Chicken is an excellent source of niacin, providing 97 percent of the RDA in just four ounces. Minerals found in chicken include selenium, zinc, copper, magnesium, phosphorus, and heme iron.

What many people don't realize is that poultry is also incredibly high in omega-6, and well-raised poultry can be much more difficult to source than red meat and fish. We are not against eating chicken and turkey, but in general, red meat and fish are more nutrient dense and have less omega-6, and it's just easier to source the good stuff.

FISH

Wild-caught fish is one of the best sources of the highly anti-inflammatory omega-3 fats, DHA, and EPA. These two types of fats are not found in plants, although some plants do contain ALA, a less-active source of omega-3s.

Fish is also high in vitamin A and is one of the few food sources of vitamin D. Fish, like other types of animal protein, is high in many B vitamins. Minerals found in fish include potassium, zinc, selenium, and iodine.

SHELLFISH

Shellfish, including foods like lobster, oysters, scallops, clams, shrimp, snails, crabs, mussels, and squid, are also an excellent source of protein and many vitamins and minerals, especially zinc. Like many other protein sources, they contain B vitamins, particularly B12. They are also high in phosphorus, potassium, iodine, and selenium.[6]

INSECT PROTEINS

We're intrigued by the growing number of insect protein companies on the market, but still not convinced that the public will accept them as a major staple of our diet. From a sustainability perspective, we're also not seeing how they are regenerating our soil, because most of these companies appear to feed their insects GMO grains. Perhaps the biggest benefit insect proteins will have on our food system is actually as an addition to chicken and pork feed, not through direct human consumption by Western populations.

ORGAN MEATS

Organ meats are the organs of animals that can be consumed as food, and used to be highly valued for their nutritional content. Common organ meats include liver, tongue, heart, brain, sweetbreads, kidneys, and tripe. Many of these organs are incredibly high in vitamins and minerals. Organ meats are high in vitamin B12, folate, and iron. They are also extremely high in fat-soluble vitamins such as vitamins A, D, E, and K. The nutritional content can vary depending on the type of meat.

IS GRASS-FED BEEF HEALTHIER THAN TYPICAL BEEF?

This is a topic that will ruffle some feathers, and has definitely started some heated arguments both online and at conferences, but it has to be said: we don't have the data to support the statement that grass-finished beef is significantly healthier for humans to eat than a typical steak. There is simply not great evidence *right now* to support the claims being made in favor of grass-fed beef *from a human nutrition standpoint.* We know, this is a shocker, but at the same time we feel that it's critical that we analyze all the available data and not cherry-pick studies that support our ideological claims.

In the largest study to date, researchers from Michigan State University analyzed the nutritional content of 750 samples of commercially available grass-fed beef loin from twelve producers across ten states in the US.[7] The beef was supplied by farms raising as few as twenty-five head and as many as 5,000 head of cattle.

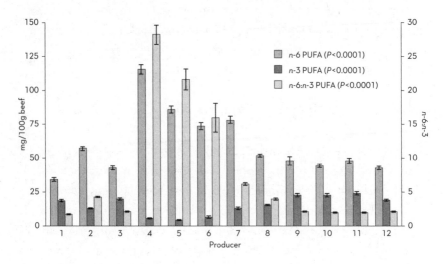

Adapted from *Meat and Muscle Biology.*

The total fat content of the beef varied widely, from 0.08 to 3.6 grams per 100 grams of beef, with an average of 0.7 grams. Comparatively, a conventional beef loin steak trimmed of all fat contains 5.6 grams of fat per 100 grams of beef.[8] There were also notable variations in the concentrations of all tested individual fatty acids. You can see the differences between grass-fed and conventional beef fat composition in the table below.

Grass-fed vs. conventional beef loin fatty acid composition (mg per 100g beef)			
Fatty acid	Grass-fed average	Grass-fed range	Conventional
Total	720	84–3,610	5,670
Saturated	320	29–1,790	2,345

Monounsaturated	320	15–1,710	2,710
Polyunsaturated	80	25–224	380
Omega-6	67	17–220	320
Linoleic acid	47	12–168	250
Arachidonic acid	17	4–50	46
CLA	1.5	0.05–23	22
Omega-3	14	1–48	20
Alpha-linolenic acid	6	0.3–30	10
EPA	3.5	0.2–14	2
DPA	4	0.4–10	8
DHA	0.3	0.05–1	0
Omega-6 to -3 ratio	9.9	1–96	16

There is a lot that can be said about the differences in fat composition, but some key claims are as follows:

- Grass-fed beef is leaner.
- Both have a similar concentration of saturated fat (45 percent of total fat).
- The ratio of omega-6 to omega-3 is far lower in grass-fed beef.
- Conventional beef provides more CLA.

Of the four major points above, the only one of real merit is that grass-fed beef is leaner. That five-gram difference in total fat content translates to 45 calories per 100 grams of beef, which can easily add up for someone eating a lot of beef and who has a low energy requirement. Still, one could just opt for leaner cuts of conventional beef such as eye of round, which has 2.5 grams of fat per 100 grams of beef.[9]

We know many may point toward the lower ratio of omega-6 to omega-3 as evidence of superiority, but look at the absolute amounts. If you eat a kilogram of beef (2.2lbs), then you are still getting only 3.2 grams of omega-6 fatty acids in conventional beef. That's three times less than the quantity supplied by an ounce of walnuts[10] and roughly equivalent to an ounce of almonds.[11] Same deal with the omega-3 content. A kilogram of grass-fed beef provides only 35 milligrams of EPA and 3 milligrams of DHA, with most of its omega-3 content being alpha-linoleic acid. One need only eat about 3 grams of chinook salmon to obtain the same amount of EPA and DHA; a 100-gram fillet provides roughly 1 gram of each.[12] And we may as well ignore the ALA since it is not readily converted into EPA and DHA—the long-chain omega-3 fatty acids associated with health benefits.[13]

That said, swapping out 690 grams per week (about 24oz) of red meat from conventional cattle for red meat from grass-fed cattle and lamb has been shown to significantly increase serum concentrations of total omega-3 fatty acids, including DHA, and reduce the ratio of serum omega-6 to omega-3.[14] Daily intake of DHA was shown to increase by 4.5 milligrams from 9.5 to 14 milligrams, which is in line with the values of DHA found in grass-fed beef.[15] However, given the wide variation in the omega-3 content of commercially available grass-fed beef samples, you have no way of knowing whether eating grass-fed beef would have the same impact on you. Plus, partici-pant screening excluded anyone who ate oily fish more than twice a month. Would eating grass-fed beef be of any note if one ate even just one serving of oily fish every week? We need to look at how a food will have an impact on the person's entire week of meals, not one bite.

The same is true regarding the CLA content. In one randomized controlled trial, having adults supplement their diet with 2.2–2.7 grams of CLA per day for several weeks had no significant effects on health markers other than a marginal reduction in triglycerides.[16] To obtain this level of CLA intake would require eating 10–12 kilo-grams (22–27lbs) of conventional beef and an equivalent amount of grass-fed beef if we use the maximum recorded CLA content (23mg per 100g of beef).

Now, many of these differences are probably quite appreciable when using isolated tallow, since it is pure fat. However, when opt-ing for beef, especially lean beef, there isn't that big of a difference between grass-fed and conventional cattle. So, when folks report that grass-finished beef has more omega-3 or CLA or whatever, we need some context for that statement. Three pennies are more than one penny, but it's still not a lot of money! The Michigan State University study also looked at concentrations of minerals and antioxidants. Again, there was wide variation in many of these compounds, including iron, zinc, copper, selenium, vitamin E, and beta-carotene. On average, amounts of most were higher than conventional beef,[17] but not to an appreciable extent. The differences amounted to roughly 1 milligram iron, 13 milligrams magnesium, 200 milligrams potassium, 20 milligrams copper, and 0.4 milligram of vitamin E.

Let's put this idea in the context of one's overall diet. Imagine someone is eating a ton of ultraprocessed foods, loaded with omega-6, where about 70 percent of intake is from grain-based foods. They eat few vegetables and no fatty fish. This is your typical American diet, where the ratio of omega-6 to -3 is likely somewhere around 20:1. Swapping typical beef for grass-fed beef in the context of that overall crappy diet is not really going to make a huge impact on their health. Now compare this to someone eating a nutrient-dense diet rich in vegetables, seafood, and meat with little to no processed foods. Let's guess this diet has a ratio of omega 6- to -3 of about 3:1. Having that person eat one more serving of salmon or sardines would have a much higher impact on omega-3 intake than switching to 100 percent grass-fed beef. We need to look at how a food will impact the person's entire week of meals, not one bite.

In short, there are differences between grass-fed and conventional beef, with grass-fed possibly being more nutritionally dense, but the impact this would have on your body is unknown. We're just not seeing consistency in the literature about nutrients in grass-fed beef or its impacts on human health. To put it another way, say we told you some studies (but not all) showed that organic carrots have twice as much protein as typical carrots. Is this the best reason to eat carrots? Who eats carrots for protein? Nutritionally, there are other reasons why folks eat carrots. There are also good environmental reasons to choose organic carrots, but is it right to tell people who can't access organic produce not to eat carrots at all?

But what about other nonnutrient constituents like pathogenic bacteria and toxicants? According to the Centers for Disease Control (CDC), in 2017 food poisoning outbreaks were most often caused by mollusks (19 percent), fish (17 percent), chicken (11 percent), and beef (9 percent).[18] For beef, the issue stems largely from *E. coli* O157:H7, which often makes its way into beef through contamination with fecal matter. Yet fecal samples of grass-fed and conventional cattle show similar concentrations of *E. coli*.[19] However, this ignores the production methods of retail beef. Consumer Reports found that *E. coli* and other pathogenic bacteria were more prevalent on commercial cuts of conventional beef than grass-fed beef,[20] likely owing to how the cattle are slaughtered and brought to market (e.g., meat and fat coming from multiple animals and slaughter rates of a couple of hundred head per hour). Plus, the bacteria on conventional cattle demonstrate a greater resistance to common antibiotics,[21] meaning that any food poisoning has a chance of being more severe. Of course, this entire issue is circumvented by simply cooking your meat enough, but that runs into other problems with palatability and the formation of carcinogens from cooking meat harshly (e.g., "well-done" or grilling).

Antibiotic resistance and its threat to human health is a significant concern, but there seems to be very little evidence that the meat you buy at the grocery store will have antibiotic residue on it. The issue with antibiotics and livestock really seems to be when drugs important to humans are overused and pass through the animal into the environment. The "antibiotic-free" label is not approved by the USDA, has no clear meaning, and doesn't necessarily mean the animal doesn't carry antibiotic-resistant bacteria. Sick livestock are treated with antibiotics but must wait for the drugs to clear before processing. The other use of antibiotics in the livestock industry is to prevent disease and promote growth. As of 2017, however, the FDA no longer allowed medically important drugs to be used in livestock for production purposes, and the livestock industry's use of those drugs is declining fast overall.[22] Any meat found positive for antibiotic residue is discarded. In 2018, less than 0.5 percent of meat sampled by the US Residue Program contained detectable amounts of antibiotics.[23] Some studies have shown more concerning amounts of antibiotic residue on meat samples in other countries[24]; however, each country has its own regulations. All meat imports to the US are inspected by the United States Department of Agriculture Food Safety Inspection Service and it is against the law for anyone to sell any meat containing unsafe levels of antibiotics. Because of the risk of drug-resistant antibiotics in the environment, we feel there's a good case to avoid industrially raised meat, but it seems that the case is less of a nutrition argument. In short, it seems quite unlikely that you'll consume antibiotic residue from typical beef, though there's a good case for better livestock management where antibiotics would be less needed. We'll cover this more in Part II.

As for toxicants, many persistent organic pollutants are lipid-soluble and stored in the fat of animals, including humans.[25] It makes sense that cattle exposed to higher levels of environmental pollutants and pesticides on their feed would contain more toxicants in their meat.[26] However, beef from cattle who eat feed grown with glyphosate show the same negligible concentrations of glyphosate as beef from cattle who never ate glyphosate.[27] Glyphosate in the feed of cattle doesn't even appear to negatively affect their body composition or metabolic health.[28] Certainly, there exists a risk that other toxicants do present in greater concentrations in beef from conventional cattle, but we don't have any evidence of this.

Another area where we don't have much research is on the effects of stress, particularly the stress occurring soon before slaughter, on the nutritional quality of meat. We've known since at least the '70s that stress within forty-eight hours of slaughter causes glucocorticoids to infiltrate the meat, lowering its pH (makes it more acidic) and making it less tender.[29] However, whether slaughter stress or chronic stress from the factory farm environment has an impact on the nutritional content of beef hasn't been investigated.

We wish that a better nutritional case for grass-fed beef could be made, as it certainly would make a simple, buttoned-up story. There is a big nutritional difference between pastured and conventional dairy, and the same goes for conventional and pasture-raised eggs and wild-caught and farmed fish. And, based on the available evidence, we can (and will) make a solid case for the environmental and ethical superiority of pastured meat. But when we consider the *nutritional* characteristics (protein, essential fats, minerals, and vitamins) alone, the delta between pastured and conventional beef is effectively nonexistent, based on the published research we've reviewed. We looked for *any* way to spin the nutrition argument in favor of grass-fed meat, but the actual data are fairly easy to verify. If we whitewashed this for a more palatable narrative, the obvious flaw in that position might cast doubt on everything else we are suggesting.

We realize that this is a remarkably unpopular position. But, going back to our carrot example, an ethical clinician would never tell a patient that they should eat only organic vegetables or no vegetables at all. We have the same position on meat. For those who simply don't have access to grass-fed beef, we still feel red meat in general is an important, nutrient-dense food for humans. We'll explore this in more detail in the next section and in chapter fifteen. In short, we applaud those who can eat only grass-fed beef, but we feel it's unethical to demand people living on a low income remove meat from their diets and replace it with less-nutritious options, which have their own environmental impacts. As parents and nutrition experts, our advice is that those who want to give their families and themselves the best advantage should feed them beef. Not everyone has the privilege to "know their farmer."

Now, before you throw out this book, this doesn't mean that we are arguing against buying grass-fed meat or saying that the science is settled on this topic. We definitely need more research. We may learn that the type of forage cattle are finished on is key, or that other compounds like polyphenols play an important role. We hope to learn more soon. There *are* certainly many other very good reasons to eat grass-finished beef, as we'll explain in the environmental and ethics sections, but nutrition (from the peer-reviewed evidence we have to date) really isn't one of them.

BUT WAIT, GOOD MEAT IS EXPENSIVE!

When people switch from a diet full of grains and processed foods to one higher in animal proteins, there is often some sticker shock. A diet higher in fresh vegetables and animal proteins is definitely more expensive than what a typical Western diet contains, and yes, grass-finished beef is pricier than typical beef.

Even so, let's look at the price of grass-finished beef versus a popular meat-free protein alternative. When we compared the prices of organic, grass-fed beef and the ultraprocessed meat alternative Beyond Burger in May 2019, the Beyond Burgers were almost twice as expensive per pound. When you compare the average price of organic grass-fed beef it's still less expensive (and more nutrient dense) than highly processed plant-based protein products. We're not seeing many people saying that tofurkey is too expensive! Per ounce, organic grass-finished beef is cheaper than many common foods like potato chips, red wine, name-brand cookies, popular coffee drinks, fancy donuts, and even fresh strawberries. And if we were to compare price per gram of protein, or per micronutrient, we'd see an even better value. There are ways to make eating real food less expensive by preparing more ground and organ meats, which are even higher in nutrients than muscle cuts. Visit Sacredcow.info for more info on sourcing and preparing meat.

In addition, we think that if more people started buying grass-fed beef, we'd see the price go down. Organic produce used to be much more expensive than it is today, and this is the result of consumer demand. In 2017 organic food sales totaled nearly $50 billion. When you compare foods according to high-quality protein and micronutrient content, the winner is clear.

But that's not where we're spending our food dollars. We're spending more on hyperpalatable, ultraprocessed foods than ever before. Intake of grains, industrially processed seed oils, and sweeteners is on the rise. On average, we spend the largest percentage of our food dollars on restaurants, and when we're out, most people eat much more and make less healthy choices than when we're home. In 2017, 53 percent of our food dollars were spent on eating out.[30]

After our spending on eating out, the majority of our food dollars are going to so-called miscellaneous foods, a category that includes premade meals, condiments, and processed snack foods like potato chips. The second most popular category is beverages, which includes soda, fruit juice, coffee, and tea, followed by bakery products, which means bread, doughnuts, cakes, and cookies. Most of what we buy is not even things we need to cook, and spending in these categories is growing every year. More people hate cooking than ever before; in fact, only 10 percent of Americans report "liking" to cook.[31]

HOW MUCH AMERICANS SPEND ON FOOD ANNUALLY ($7,023 AVERAGE)

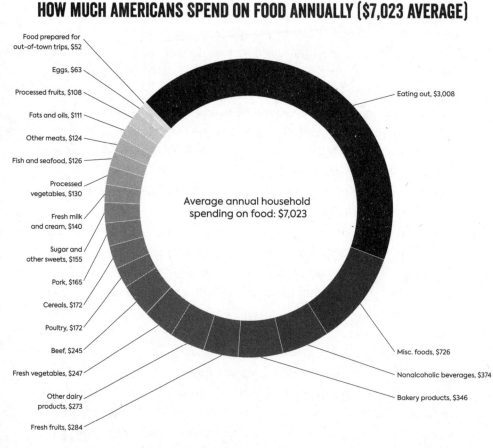

Food prepared for out-of-town trips, $52
Eggs, $63
Processed fruits, $108
Fats and oils, $111
Other meats, $124
Fish and seafood, $126
Processed vegetables, $130
Fresh milk and cream, $140
Sugar and other sweets, $155
Pork, $165
Cereals, $172
Poultry, $172
Beef, $245
Fresh vegetables, $247
Other dairy products, $273
Fresh fruits, $284

Eating out, $3,008

Average annual household spending on food: $7,023

Misc. foods, $726
Nonalcoholic beverages, $374
Bakery products, $346

Sources: Business Insider[32] and the Bureau of Labor Statistics.

These modern hyperpalatable foods bypass our brain's natural appetite regulation system and thus contribute to overeating. These foods tick most of the boxes we'd associate with addictive substances such as cocaine and opiates. Some would argue that anything meeting these parameters should be heavily regulated, perhaps banned or heavily taxed. But from what we've seen historically, prohibition doesn't do much in the way of mitigating intake of addictive substances. It's outside the scope of this book to thoroughly dig into the economics of the junk food industry, but we would like to humbly suggest that perhaps the government should not be in the business of making junk food cheap, and if we as a society do decide to tax junk foods such as soda, we should certainly not tax it while continuing to subsidize the production of its main ingredients.

Whatever good intentions the subsidies programs may have started under, government subsidies of junk food are not doing consumers any favors. Let's look at a little home economics. A quick Amazon search reveals a ten-count box of Hostess Twinkies for $4.67, which is about what you'd find them for in most supermarkets. This puts the price of these delectable little morsels at forty-seven cents for each Twinkie. The price for organic apples (in season when they are cheapest) is about $2.99 per pound. Each apple weighs about one-third of a pound, which puts organic apples at just about a dollar each. Now, we didn't look at organic apples to be hoity-toity, but because most organic produce and grass-fed meat does not receive *any* government subsidies, the price you see reflects real market-based supply and demand.

On one level that Twinkie appears cheap, but let's look at how much this is costing in terms of the energy we get from each product: the Twinkie provides 160 calories, mainly in the form of refined flour, sugar, and vegetable oils (all items that are so cheap largely because of subsidies). The apple, by contrast, is about 95 calories, mainly from a mix of sugars, but it also provides a hefty dose of fiber, antioxidants, vitamins, and minerals. Let's see how these two items play out with regards to calories per dollar.

Apple: 95 calories per dollar
Twinkie: 347 calories per dollar

For all the talk about privilege in our modern dialogue, we don't seem to talk enough about the fact that the cheapest foods are often the unhealthiest, which has a disproportionate effect where people can't spend as much on food (low-income neighborhoods, communities of color, and rural areas).[33] For people living at the margins, it is clear one may obtain more total calories for less money by eating unhealthy food. Yet when we talk about fulfilling human nutritional needs, we obviously can't look at meeting our calorie needs alone. We also need to think about getting the right nutrients, and the most nutrient-dense food these groups (or anyone) could eat—namely, meat—is unfairly criticized as unhealthy.

This is where the "less meat, better meat" ideology can be problematic when we consider the public health impacts of this message. We don't hear people say "organic vegetables or no vegetables" or "less vegetables, better vegetables." Many people don't have access to grass-finished beef, or can't afford it; there are manifold benefits to eating more protein, specifically from animal sources like beef; and there are few human health advantages to eating grass-finished beef compared to typical beef. So our position is that folks should buy the best meat they can afford. A burger made from feedlot finished beef is still a better choice, from a caloric and nutrient-density perspective, than junk food (or, as we'll see in the next chapter, even beans and rice). If we are to solve our growing obesity and diabetes issues, the message of "less meat" is not going to help.

CHAPTER 6

EVEN IF MEAT ISN'T BAD FOR ME, CAN'T I GET ALL MY NUTRITION FROM PLANTS?

We feel that we've made a pretty good case for the health benefits of meat, but some folks might still not want to eat it for other reasons. We'll walk you through our environmental and ethical case for better meat soon, but let's first talk about why diets that exclude all animal products are not optimal.

Let's back up for a minute and look at the different forms of "meat-free" diets. There's a huge difference in the nutritional impact depending on the amount of animal products consumed. And the term "vegetarian" can mean different things. Pesco-pollo vegetarians avoid red meat and eat plants, chicken, and fish. Pescatarians eat only plants and fish and exclude chicken or beef. Lacto-ovo vegetarians eat vegetables plus dairy products and eggs. Vegans exclude all animal products completely. The types of food included or excluded in each of these diets vary greatly. Vegetarians who eat dairy and eggs are actually consuming animal products, so we must treat them very differently from vegans who eat *only* plants. It's much easier to be healthy and feel full with the high-quality proteins and fats that eggs and dairy provide. We see fewer health complications, like nutrient deficiencies, with vegetarians when compared to vegans. For our purposes in this chapter, we'll define *vegetarian* as a diet that includes eggs and dairy but no meat, poultry, or fish, and *vegan* as a diet that avoids all animal products.

If one was to design a well-balanced diet without *any* animal products, it would focus on low-glycemic vegetables and protein mostly from soaked legumes; it would not include fake meats or other highly processed foods. With some effort, and a lot of supplements, this could be a nutritious diet for *some* people; however, we don't have data on how this diet works over several generations of mothers and their children. As we'll discuss, we disagree that a totally plant-based diet is best for all people, and indeed, it may even be unsafe for some.

NOT ALL PROTEIN IS THE SAME

We've already explained that the most common recommendations for daily protein intake are lower than what we consider optimal. Protein is much more difficult to get from plants than from animals, and vegetarians and vegans can more easily be protein deficient than people who eat meat and poultry.

Protein is made up of amino acids (AAs). There are twenty AAs that our bodies utilize, nine of which are essential, meaning that our bodies must obtain these from food. (By contrast, a "nonessential" nutrient doesn't mean we don't need it; it simply means that our bodies can make it from the building blocks in other nutrients, so we don't require it directly from our diets. That being said, conversion can be a difficult process, so consuming the true form is always preferred.) Animal products contain all the AAs we need, while plants lack one or more AAs, particularly leucine, which is one of the most important AAs for humans. So when a package of food lists "grams of protein," it doesn't really give you the full story on the spectrum of amino acids or how digestible the protein is by humans.

The protein quality in animal products is very different than the protein quality in plants. There are a couple of different ways that researchers and health professionals measure protein quality. The protein digestibility-corrected amino acid score (PDCAAS) was introduced in 1989 by the Food and Agriculture Organization and World Health Organization and has been widely adopted as the preferred method for measuring how proteins best meet human nutrition needs. The table below, with data from the *Journal of Sports Science & Medicine*, shows beef, casein, eggs, milk, soy, and whey proteins as the highest in nutritional value by PDCAAS.[1]

Protein Type	Protein Digestibility-Corrected Amino Acid Score
Casein	1.00
Egg	1.00
Milk	1.00
Soy protein	1.00
Whey protein	1.00
Beef	0.92
Black beans	0.75
Peanuts	0.52
Wheat gluten	0.25

However, the PDCAAS does not account for antinutritional factors like trypsin inhibitors, lectins, and tannins, which can reduce protein hydrolysis and amino acid absorption from plant-based proteins like soy (we will talk about this soon).[2] Digestibility of plant proteins is also affected by age and the state of the person's gut.[3] It is widely agreed that animal protein (eggs, milk, meat, fish, and poultry) is the most bioavailable source.[4] Meat-based proteins also have no limiting amino acids, whereas soy is low in the AA methionine and is not considered a "complete" protein.

Let's compare beans and beef. As you can see from the tables that follow, which contain data from the USDA's nutrient database, four ounces of cooked kidney beans not only has far less protein than the same amount of sirloin steak but is also much lower in vitamins and minerals, making beef far more nutrient dense per calorie than beans.

Of course, kidney beans and sirloin steak are just two examples, but animal products overall are a much better source of protein per calorie than plants. For example, to get 30 grams of protein, you could eat about 137 calories worth of fish, 181 calories of steak, or *640 calories* of beans (which adds an additional 122 grams of carbohydrate). This doesn't necessarily mean you should never eat beans and rice, but it certainly illustrates that if we're trying to reduce overall calories and limit carbs, plant-based proteins are not the solution.

BEEF VS BEANS - PROTEIN

Animal sources are the **most complete protein sources** because they contain all of the amino acids we need for **optimal health**. To get the same amount of protein in a 4oz steak (181 calories) you'd need to eat **12oz of kidney beans plus a cup of rice**, which equals **638 calories, and 122g of carbs.**

4oz SIRLOIN STEAK

Total Protein = 30g

Amino Acid	Amount	% DRI
Cystine	0.4g	59%
Histidine	1.3g	147%
Isoleucine	1.6g	135%
Leucine	3.0g	113%
Lysine	3.4g	138%
Methionine	0.9g	156%
Phenylaline	1.4g	133%
Threonine	1.6g	129%
Tryptophan	0.4g	123%
Tyrosine	1.3g	124%
Valine	1.7g	114%

181	30g	0g	4.5g
Calories	Protein	Carbs	Fat

4oz KIDNEY BEANS

Total Protein = 9g

Amino Acid	Amount	% DRI
Cystine	0.1g	15%
Histidine	0.3g	30%
Isoleucine	0.5g	38%
Leucine	0.8g	31%
Lysine	0.7g	28%
Methionine	0.1g	21%
Phenylaline	0.6g	55%
Threonine	0.4g	28%
Tryptophan	0.1g	37%
Tyrosine	0.2g	22%
Valine	0.6g	37%

144	9g	18.4g	0.6g
Calories	Protein	Carbs	Fat

BEEF VS BEANS - VITAMINS

Steak is more **nutrient dense** than beans, especially when it comes to B vitamins. A 4oz piece of steak meets **95% of the DRI for B12**, one of the most common nutrient deficiencies worldwide.

4oz SIRLOIN STEAK

		% DRI
B1 (Thiamine)	0.1mg	8%
B2 (Riboflavin)	0.3mg	30%
B3 (Niacin)	9.0mg	64%
B5 (Pantothenic A.)	0.5mg	10%
B6 Pyridoxine	0.9mg	68%
B12 (Cobalamin)	2.3µg	95%
Folate	5.7µg	1%
Vitamin A	15.9 IU	1%
Vitamin C	0.0g	0%
Vitamin D	1.1 IU	0%
Vitamin E	0.3mg	2%
Vitamin K	2.2µg	2%

181	30g	0g	4.5g
Calories	Protein	Carbs	Fat

4oz KIDNEY BEANS

		% DRI
B1 (Thiamine)	0.2mg	16%
B2 (Riboflavin)	0.1mg	6%
B3 (Niacin)	0.7mg	5%
B5 (Pantothenic A.)	0.2mg	5%
B6 Pyridoxine	0.1mg	10%
B12 (Cobalamin)	0.0µg	0%
Folate	147.4µg	37%
Vitamin A	0.0 IU	0%
Vitamin C	1.4mg	2%
Vitamin D	1.1 IU	0%
Vitamin E	0.0mg	0%
Vitamin K	2.5µg	11%

144	9g	18.4g	0.6g
Calories	Protein	Carbs	Fat

BEEF VS BEANS - MINERALS

A 4oz piece of steak provides **more than half** the DRI of zinc and selenium, and is a good source of phosphorus. Overall, beef is **more nutrient dense** than beans per serving.

4oz SIRLOIN STEAK

		% DRI
Calcium	18.1mg	2%
Copper	0.1mg	7%
Iron	3.3mg	18%
Magnesium	17.0mg	5%
Manganese	0.0mg	0%
Phosphorus	306.2mg	44%
Potassium	435.4mg	9%
Selenium	30.8µg	56%
Sodium	76.0mg	3%
Zinc	5.1mg	64%

181	30g	0g	4.5g
Calories	Protein	Carbs	Fat

4oz KIDNEY BEANS

		% DRI
Calcium	39.7mg	4%
Copper	0.2mg	27%
Iron	2.5mg	14%
Magnesium	47.6mg	15%
Manganese	0.5mg	27%
Phosphorus	156.5mg	22%
Potassium	459.3mg	10%
Selenium	1.2µg	2%
Sodium	1.1mg	0%
Zinc	1.1mg	14%

144	9g	18.4g	0.6g
Calories	Protein	Carbs	Fat

CALORIES NEEDED TO GET 30 GRAMS PROTEIN

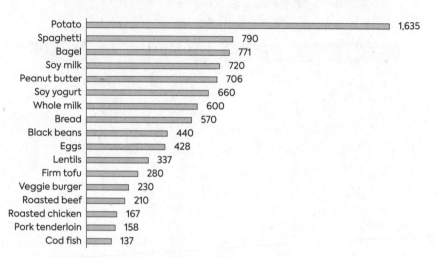

Food	Calories
Potato	1,635
Spaghetti	790
Bagel	771
Soy milk	720
Peanut butter	706
Soy yogurt	660
Whole milk	600
Bread	570
Black beans	440
Eggs	428
Lentils	337
Firm tofu	280
Veggie burger	230
Roasted beef	210
Roasted chicken	167
Pork tenderloin	158
Cod fish	137

Again, if we're aiming for 20 percent of a 2,000-calorie diet to come from protein, that is 100 grams.

Let's look at how this difference between plant and animal protein translates into public dietary advice. In an effort to simplify how Americans can get their protein, "my plate" recommendations are intended to break down the US Dietary Guidelines into "simple" terms and to be used as a mass teaching tool. The USDA has broken down protein foods into "protein equivalents," and unfortunately, if one were to follow this advice and try to get one's protein from plant sources, one would certainly come up short. Here are protein equivalents in the animal-versus-plant category:

Animal Sources		
1oz cooked beef	8.3g protein	53 calories
1oz cooked ham	5.9g protein	41 calories
1oz cooked chicken	8.8g protein	49 calories
1 sandwich slice of turkey	4.9g protein	31 calories
1oz cooked fish or shellfish	6.5g protein	30 calories
1 egg	6.3g protein	78 calories

Plant Sources		
0.5oz almonds	6g protein	164 calories
0.5oz pumpkin seeds	8.5g protein	163 calories
1 tablespoon peanut butter	3.6g protein	96 calories
¼ cup cooked black beans	3.5g protein	60 calories
¼ cup cooked chickpeas	3.6g protein	67 calories
¼ cup baked beans or refried beans	3g protein	60 calories
¼ cup (about 2oz) tofu	6.8g protein	68 calories
1oz cooked tempeh	5.6g protein	55 calories
¼ cup roasted soybeans	10g protein	104 calories
2 tablespoons hummus	2.2g protein	53 calories

As you can see, meat and seafood are much more efficient ways to get your protein compared to plant-based sources. The soy products are the closest options to animal protein, but soy is problematic, as we'll describe soon. Most of us are not looking to increase our caloric consumption, yet we want to feel full. Increasing protein is a great way to do this; animal sources are the most desirable sources, in terms of bioavailable protein *and* other micronutrients.

With the increasing interest in "clean" alternative fats, milks, and plant-based proteins, it's critical that we acknowledge that they're not nutritionally equal to the real thing. Almond milk, although it's a white liquid, pales in nutritional content to actual milk. Plant-based burgers and lab meat are not "real food." Some of these alternatives may seem similar to the real thing on the nutrition panel of the package, but as we've shown, plant-based protein is not the same as animal-based protein in terms of amino acids, and enriching a product with synthetic vitamins and minerals doesn't mean we will absorb them in the same way we do from natural sources. These products are popularly seen as "healthier" and better options than meat, but are actually ultraprocessed foods, and often much worse for our health than the real thing.

If you're happy with your health, weight, and metabolism on a plant-based diet, then fantastic. If you're not, then please consider pulling in some animal protein to help cut down on calories, help you feel satiated, and give you a boost of vital nutrients you are likely lacking.*

WHY EAT PLANTS?

If meat is so great, why do we need to eat anything from the plant kingdom? There are a growing number of folks who seem to be thriving on the carnivore diet (only animal products), believe it or not (check out the work of Shawn Baker, MD, whose book and website show people having great success with a meat-focused diet). While this seems quite promising for those who have severe food intolerances and shouldn't be ruled out as a therapeutic tool, most people do enjoy and benefit from eating plant foods. As you'll see in the "Eat Like a Nutrivore" section, we are certainly not pushing for everyone to adopt a meat-only diet! Fruits and vegetables taste good, are generally low in calories, and contain useful nutrients like vitamins, minerals, antioxidants, fats, and protein. But plants can be quite difficult to digest and have defenses that can block nutrient absorption. There are ways to make plants more digestible through cooking and fermentation, but we feel strongly that plants alone cannot meet our nutritional needs.

Although animal products contain the richest sources of most micronutrients required by humans, there are some vitamins and minerals that are best found in plants—for example, vitamins folate, C, E, and betaine. In the mineral category, plants provide greater quantities of magnesium, potassium, selenium, and manganese than most animal sources.

It's worth noting that on paper, foods like lettuce can appear to have a high nutrient-density score. This is because on a *per-calorie* basis they can contain a lot of vitamins and minerals. But once we factor in the volume of food and the number of calories in a typical

---

* We have a long, detailed blog post taking a critical look at amino acids in plant foods versus animal foods at www.sacredcow.info/blog/are-all-proteins-created-equal.

serving size, the picture changes very quickly. One cup of lettuce has only eight calories, so the volume of lettuce you'd need to eat to match the same nutrient-density in a small serving of, say, oysters is quite dramatic.

Nuts and seeds are an excellent source of minerals, including magnesium, manganese, copper, selenium, and zinc. But relying only on nuts as your primary source of these minerals can have a few downsides. Most nuts are high in omega-6 fats, which are already found in excess in many of our diets and compete for absorption of anti-inflammatory omega-3s. We do need some omega-6 fats for health, but most of us are already eating too much, so adding an additional source of omega-6 may not be ideal.[5] They also contain antinutrients (see the next section).

Although plants contain calcium, bioavailability of calcium from food can vary greatly. Even soybeans, which are considered "high" in calcium, are only 30–40 percent bioavailable. Soy milk, which is frequently used as an alternative to cow's milk, is fortified with calcium, increasing the bioavailability to 75 percent. Although many of these plant foods do contain calcium, the amount absorbed is quite low.[6] Nonheme iron comes from plant sources and is not as well absorbed as iron from animal protein, as it is not bound to any protein. Iron absorption from plants is low, at about 5–12 percent.[7]

Plants contain the pigment beta-carotene and phytochemicals, which have beneficial antioxidant properties.[8] Herbs like peppermint, spices like cloves, espresso, red wine, and dark chocolate are noted for their high antioxidant content.[9] It's common to see supplements containing high doses of antioxidants lining the shelves of health food stores, but they can be dangerous in high levels.[10] Most of these vitamins are manufactured in a few chemical plants in China and then sprayed on processed foods to prevent deficiency as opposed to the broad spectrum of antioxidants and vitamins found in natural foods.[11]

ANTINUTRIENTS

All living creatures need a way to defend themselves against being killed or eaten so they can spread their genes into the next generation. Unlike animals, plants are unable to run away. They need another way to protect themselves from insects and other animals that consume them. Therefore, they have created other types of defenses in order to attempt to produce offspring. While many plants are downright poisonous to humans, others will do their best to use you as a vehicle to spread their seeds, sending out chemical defenses while they pass through your intestines. (Those of you who have eaten corn on the cob may have noticed that those corn kernels make it through surprisingly intact.)

These chemical defenses found in plants are referred to as antinutrients. They can be found in roots, leaves, and seeds. Some are bitter substances that discourage animals from eating that plant again.

Antinutrients are found in the largest quantities in cereals and legumes, although they can be in other plants also.

Common antinutrients include the following:

- Saponins
- Phytic acid (phytate)
- Gluten
- Tannins
- Oxalates
- Lectins
- Polyphenols
- Flavonoids
- Trypsin inhibitors
- Isoflavones
- Solanine
- Chaconine[12]

One of the primary problems with antinutrients is that, as their name implies, they work "against" nutrients. They can prevent nutrient absorption by binding to vitamins and minerals, which may lead to nutritional deficiencies. They can also prevent the absorption of protein, in the case of legumes, which may lead to protein deficiency if the diet is not well balanced to include other protein sources. Certain antinutrients are enzyme inhibitors that interfere with the function of important digestive enzymes, leading to gastrointestinal problems. Some are so poisonous that the toxins can accumulate to a level where cell and tissue functions are disrupted.

Phytic acid, for example, has been found to significantly reduce absorption of zinc, iron, and calcium—and those minerals might be the exact reason we are eating these specific foods! Phytic acid does this by interfering with the enzymes that break down these foods during digestion in order to extract these important minerals. Some phytic acid can be removed from grains, nuts, and seeds by soaking and roasting, but it is unclear how much remains and the effect on absorption.[13]

Iron deficiency can be a particular challenge in meat-free diets because oxalates, tannins, and phytates all block iron absorption. For example, many people think that spinach is a great source of iron, but only 2 percent of the iron in spinach is actually absorbed. This is because it's a nonheme form, but also because spinach is high in oxalates, which block iron absorption.[14] Oxalates also reduce calcium bioavailability; in spinach, it is reduced to just 5 percent, even though spinach does have a lot of calcium.

However, antinutrients are not all bad. For example, flavonoids are considered an antinutrient, but they have many health benefits owing to their function as antioxidants. Even though antinutrients may at times interfere with vitamin and mineral absorption or may make certain people ill, most people should be able to tolerate some amount of foods that contain antinutrients, especially when these foods are prepared properly.

THE PROBLEMS WITH SOY

Soy is one of the few plant foods that provides all nine essential amino acids, so it is often promoted as an amazing alternative to meat. But there is a troubling amount of research linking soy to digestive problems, reproductive issues, and cognitive decline.

A big reason soy intake is subject to so much research and controversy is because soy is high in antinutrients, particularly isoflavones. These plant compounds are similar to estrogen and are used by the soy plant as a natural defense, disrupting the reproductive cycle of livestock that eat it.[15] Some research has suggested that isoflavones could result in a disruption in fertility, hormone balance, and thyroid function in humans.[16] How these compounds behave in the body is complicated, and it's beyond the scope of this book to fully dive into all the research on soy—thousands of studies have investigated it. But we think there are a couple things to keep in mind.

Traditional cultures that consume a lot of soy-based products tend to ferment or prepare the soy in a manner that reduces the content of the antinutrients, reducing the risk of toxicity. But in most Western societies we consume soy in the form of soybean oil, soy protein isolate (a highly processed, high-protein powder), or as soy lecithin (a combination of soybean oil and phospholipids). We have already addressed how soybean oil is high in omega-6 fats, further skewing the ratio between essential fatty acids.

Soy products consumed in this highly processed form can be problematic for health. People with allergies to soy can be triggered by soy lecithin, which is hidden in foods as a common emulsifier.[17] Soy lecithin may also impair cognitive function and impact brain chemistry.[18]

Given that research has raised troubling questions about how safe soy is, we think meat is a superior option; it offers much more nutrition for the calories. Our take is that soy should be limited or avoided in the diet, especially in the forms commonly found in processed and packaged foods.

HOW TO MAKE PLANTS MORE DIGESTIBLE

Soaking, sprouting, cooking, fermenting, or even just chewing plants can help reduce their negative effects on digestion and reduce toxins to some degree. For example, cassava or yucca is a primary source of carbohydrates for people in many African countries. Cassava, if not properly processed, is high in cyanide and therefore extremely toxic. But, through a variety of preparation processes such as fermenting, drying, soaking, and cooking, the plant becomes an excellent source of concentrated carbohydrates.[19]

Although plants can be difficult to digest and some contain antinutrients, we still feel it's important to incorporate a large variety of plants in your diet, as tolerated. Eating plants raw allows for the preservation of certain enzymes, antioxidants, and water-soluble vitamins that are sensitive to heat. Cooked, fermented, and sprouted plants do allow for better digestion by breaking them down and helping inactivate antinutrients.

WHAT HAPPENS WHEN YOU GIVE UP ANIMAL PRODUCTS?

For a while it seemed like you couldn't go a week without hearing yet another celebrity went vegan. We feel that it's important to acknowledge that staying healthy while eating only plants is much easier for privileged people who have the time, knowledge, and means to do the research and purchase the necessary supplements. This ends up working out pretty well for wealthy celebrities, and not so great for infants, picky teenagers, those struggling with illness, and those less educated when it comes to nutrition requirements. We are acutely concerned for the growing number of teenagers we see going vegan because they think it's "cool." Parents whose children announce that they're giving up meat often feel compelled to support them, yet they might not know the right way to follow a vegan diet. Most parents aren't educated enough on the importance of protein and critical micronutrients to help their kids maximize their nutrition when removing animal products. Many kids and teens are picky eaters who, when they push away meat, are left with bagels, pasta, white bread, and rice as the main feature on their plates. The damages that start to quickly accrue in this situation begin with an altered gut biome and hormonal and metabolic derangement from eating so many processed carbohydrates. Teenage girls can lose their periods, experience hair loss and worsening acne, and their energy and immune systems can crash, leaving them exhausted and constantly sick. (Diana works with this population frequently, trying to reverse the damage of a poor vegan diet among teens.)

Although we'll talk about the environmental implications of meat in the next part of this book, it's important to note that a recent study looked at the nutritional and environmental implications of removing animals from US agriculture. It found that although greenhouse gas emissions would be reduced by a mere 2.6 percent, we would create a food system incapable of meeting our nutritional needs. In their plant-only system, the US would produce 23 percent more food, but we would be lacking in nutrients. A plant-only system would result in deficiencies in calcium, vitamin K, vitamin D, choline, and essential fatty acids. It would also result in a 12 percent increase in total calories.[20] Our food system doesn't have a problem producing calories (human "feed"). What we need is *nutrients*.

While it could be argued that a well-planned vegan diet could be more nutrient dense than a diet full of processed foods, neither a vegan nor a Western diet mimics what humans have traditionally eaten. When we look at traditional cultures, none of them have been 100 percent plant based. Animal products, whether it's eggs and dairy or including animal flesh of some kind, are part of every group ever studied. On the flip side, there are traditional cultures that thrived on very few to virtually no plants.

You might know people who are healthy long-term and follow a plant-based diet. As you probably already know, genetics plays a big role on how we look, our disease risk, and our life expectancy; our genes can also affect our reaction to particular foods. For example, plant foods contain an inactive form of vitamin A called beta-carotene. However, almost half the population have a gene that reduces the conversion of beta-carotene to vitamin A by approximately 70 percent.[21] Other factors that affect how someone would react to a vegan diet would be gut integrity, health status, and age.

A diet that might work for a healthy adult doesn't necessarily mean it's a good idea for babies, growing children, or the elderly.

You may run into some (new) vegans or vegetarians who claim they are thriving on this diet. They say things like "I have never been more mentally clear!" "I have lost 20 pounds!" or "I finally don't feel sick anymore." And this may be true for a time. In starting a vegetarian or vegan diet, people tend to also eliminate a lot of problematic foods like sugar and processed foods, which will immediately make *anyone* healthier. But this great feeling of health has nothing to do with the elimination of animal foods, as many would like to believe. In truth, a vegan diet can be similar to a fast. Fasts can be a good thing, *temporarily*, and fasts tend to help people feel better and improve several health markers, at least at first.[22] Vegan diets also eliminate two sources of common triggers of food intolerances: dairy and eggs. Without these foods in the diet, many people may actually feel better, have fewer digestive problems, and lose weight.

But what about the science? A lot of the studies on the benefits of eliminating meat tend to also modify several other variables in the experimental group. The researchers tend to also ask subjects to eliminate processed foods, start exercising, or implement other healthy habits on top of avoiding meat. And as we learned in chapter four, with all these changes toward a healthier lifestyle, it is impossible to determine the exact cause of the results. We simply have no proof that eliminating animal products, while keeping all other factors the same, will improve health.

Many vegetarians and vegans feel much better when initially shifting to this way of eating. But it's not for the reasons they might think; it's probably not the meat. If new vegetarians or vegans decrease their intake of junk food and increase their intake of plants, this may be a major shift from what they were eating before in terms of nutrient density. They are likely getting more vitamins, minerals, and antioxidants simply from following a whole food diet. And, in fact, removing animal products is a risky endeavor that can result in deficiencies.

NUTRIENT DEFICIENCIES IN VEGAN AND VEGETARIAN DIETS

For those following a meat-free diet, it's very easy to be low in dietary protein and other key nutrients, which can affect physical and mental health. Those who cut animal-based foods out of their diets must find alternative sources to stay healthy. Let's take a closer look at some of the more common problems.

B12 DEFICIENCY

Among the most concerning nutrient deficiencies prevalent in the vegetarian and vegan population is vitamin B12: 60 percent of adult vegans have been found to be deficient in B12,[23] as well as 40 percent of vegetarians.[24] A deficiency in B12 can cause depression, psychosis, and cognitive impairment.[25] A deficiency in B12 can lead to irreversible consequences for children, including delayed cognitive development, lower academic performance, nerve damage, and failure to thrive. Because of the severity and long-term impact of these symptoms, the Academy of Nutrition and Dietetics does recommend supplementation of B12 via fortified foods or supplements for all vegans and vegetarians. Plant foods like seaweed contain B12 analogs and not the true form of B12. These analogs actually increase your need for the true form of B12.[26] Most soy products do not contain B12. The traditional Asian soy product tempeh does (it's associated with the fermentation process), but at only 0.7–8.0 µg for every 100 grams, one would need to consume 300 grams of tempeh daily to reach the RDA of 2.4 µg a day for adult humans. That's a lot of tempeh!

IRON DEFICIENCY

Iron deficiency is the most common nutrient deficiency worldwide, affecting approximately 25 percent of the global population and almost half of all preschool children. Iron deficiency can lead to severe and chronic diseases, chronic heart failure, cancer, and inflammatory bowel disease.[27] In children it can cause serious developmental delays and behavioral issues. Vegetarians are commonly iron deficient, which is a risk factor for type 2 diabetes.[28] Heme iron, found in red meat, is the most absorbable kind of iron, two to three times better than plant-based iron, and absorption is also dependent on current iron stores. In New Zealand, hospitalizations for iron deficiency have doubled over the last ten years as red meat consumption has declined.[29] Vegetarianism in New Zealand is up nearly 30 percent, and of those who do eat meat, they're eating more than twice as much chicken and pork, yet beef and lamb consumption are dramatically down. Early signs of iron deficiency include fatigue, light-headedness, and shortness of breath. Although a package label of a meat-free food may say it contains a lot of iron, only about 1.4–7 percent of plant-based iron can actually be absorbed, compared to 20 percent in red meat.[30]

LOW CALCIUM

Vegans have been found to have higher bone turnover owing to low calcium and vitamin D, which are both critical for bone health.[31] The calcium found in plant foods is not as bioavailable as calcium from foods like dairy and sardines.[32] Greens like spinach and kale contain compounds that actually block calcium absorption. In fact, one study suggested that you would need to consume five to six cups of cooked spinach to get the same calcium found in a glass of milk.[33] Low calcium and vitamin D stores (another nutrient low in vegan diets)[34] are a very big concern for bone health. Fracture rates are 30 percent higher among vegans than among those who consume animal products.[35] Other nutrients of concern for those on meat-free diets include glycine, selenium, methionine, taurine, creatine, choline, and iodine.[36] Iodine deficiency can lead to brain damage and irreversible mental retardation.[37]

IMPAIRED MENTAL FUNCTION

There are several studies that have found a disturbing link between depression and meat-free diets. Many of the nutrients commonly missing in meat-free diets are directly shown to have impacts on depression and anxiety. Zinc, for example, is not easily found in plants and has been documented as low in vegans. One study supplementing with zinc for twelve weeks showed an improvement in mood.[38] The rates of EPA and DHA deficiency are also much higher in psychiatric patients and doctors have been successfully supplementing with fish oil, seeing improvements in mental health among their patients.[39] As a society, the US is already suffering from deficiencies in key nutrients best found in animal products that can interfere with brain health. For those of you who are avoiding animal products and suffer from depression or other mental health issues, this could be a great reason to incorporate some of these nutrients in their real food form to see if it helps.

COMMON DEFICIENCIES AND THEIR EFFECTS

Many of the nutrients commonly deficient in much of the US population can affect mental health, and animals provide the best source of the majority of these. The following table lists some of the more common nutrient deficiencies and the brain functions that may be affected.[40]

Nutrient	Deficiency rate in the United States	Key Brain Function
Zinc	10%	Serotonin synthesis
Vitamin B6	10%	Neurotransmitter synthesis
Vitamin D3	10%	Calcium regulation
Iron	10–20%	Neurotransmitter synthesis
Vitamin B12	25%	Myelin synthesis
Magnesium	25%	Glutamate inhibition
Omega-3 fatty acids	80%	Neural signaling

Creatine, a substance found naturally in our muscles, is lower in vegetarian diets and may also influence healthy brain development. Creatine supplementation has been shown in one study to improve cognitive performance (by a significant level) in vegetarians. Similar improvements were not seen in subjects who ate meat, suggesting that vegetarians were performing lower on the tests owing to existing low creatine levels. The results of this study suggest that a creatine deficiency may lower fluid intelligence and working memory by up to one standard deviation, approximately fifteen IQ points. The authors write,

> It is possible that, although vegetarianism appeals to people with higher intelligence, becoming vegetarian reduces fluid intelligence and working memory . . . People may not notice a reduction in cognitive functioning when they become vegetarian if fluid but not crystallized intelligence is affected. (That is to say, becoming vegetarian may impair one's ability to solve problems without causing one to forget what one has learned, so the effect may not be noticeable.)

The decrease in cognitive function was reversed with supplementation of creatine.[41] This particular study was conducted with adults, and there have not been any long-term studies on the impact of creatine intake and brain development in children, so we don't know what the effect in kids might be.

The inability to get adequate amounts of EPA and DHA, two critical omega-3 fats necessary for brain health, is another concern on a vegan diet. Some plants do provide ALA, an omega-3 that is generally poorly converted into the active forms. Certain people are able to effectively convert ALA into EPA, though the ability to do so is dependent on other nutrients, particularly zinc, iron, and pyridoxine, all of which are very difficult to get enough of when all animal products are removed.

Because many people choose to eliminate meat for environmental or ethical reasons, when there is a health decline, some people tend not to realize that the food they're eating is causing the problem. People may simply feel their health issues come from not following the diet strictly enough. And, for certain people, even taking the "right" supplements isn't enough.

In her book *The Vegetarian Myth*, Lierre Keith explains how much her body suffered because of eliminating meat. Lierre became vegan at the age of sixteen after learning about the horrors of industrial-scale animal production. She did her research and made sure her diet contained all the right combinations of proteins. She took B12 supplements, and ate lots of fruits and vegetables. Most of the protein in her diet came from soy products. She followed the diet for twenty years. Although she lost her period, suffered from depression, and developed degenerative disc disease that caused morphine-level pain, she explains that she never really drew the connection between her medical problems and her diet. Her pain became absolutely crippling, and her exhaustion unbearable. She went to see a qigong master, whom she heard had "cured the incurable." He quickly summed up her state and sympathetically told her she must eat some meat. She went to the store, picked up a can of tuna and a plastic fork (because she didn't want to contaminate her dishes), and ate it. "Oh my god, I thought: this is what it feels like to be alive. I put my head down and sobbed," she writes.

If you are someone eating mostly or all plants, and have some health issues like fatigue, light-headedness, acne, skin rashes, mood swings, brain fog, digestive distress, blood sugar regulation problems, or other health symptoms, it's critical to consider that being meat-free could be contributing to these issues. Because humans are omnivores and a vegan diet requires supplementation, which still doesn't always work, we feel that while it's one thing for an adult to choose to be vegan, imposing a meat-free diet on children can have serious consequences.*

---

* We have outlined in chapter seventeen what our recommendations are for an optimal diet template, but for a deeper dive on nutrient density, comparing meat-rich, omnivore, and vegan diets, please visit www.sacredcow.info/blog/what-if-we-all-went-plant-based.

IS A MEAT-FREE DIET SAFE FOR ALL STAGES OF LIFE?

Like all the questions we explore in the book, the following is a controversial topic—but this one might be one of the toughest. Along with the push to eliminate meat from our diets, there are a growing number of resources aimed at helping raise children vegan. Given the nutrition research we've shared in the last few chapters, it probably won't surprise you that we're strongly against this. We're trying to be sensitive to people's ethical diet considerations, but as we've just learned, it can be much, much harder to stay healthy on a vegan diet.

Growth starts with a healthy pregnancy, which allows the fetus to develop appropriately. We all know how important it is to get adequate nutrition while pregnant. And some of the most important nutrients for growing babies—protein, calcium, vitamin B12, vitamin D—are found in animal products. Even so, many resources dismiss concerns about eating vegan or vegetarian during pregnancy, saying it's fine to get these nutrients from other sources. As we've just seen, it may *not* be easy to get these nutrients without meat, eggs, or dairy, though it is possible.

It's well known that the fatty acid DHA is needed for brain development in infants. However, DHA is absent in a vegan diet without supplementation. Among vegan women, one paper found that the DHA content of their breastmilk was 69 percent lower than that of mothers who ate animal products,[42] and another study showed that babies born to vegetarian mothers had lower DHA in their blood than babies born to meat-eating moms.[43]

One of the markers of healthy pregnancies and adequate nutrition is male-to-female sex ratio; on average, there are 105 male babies born for every 100 females. Malnutrition and lack of adequate calories during pregnancy has been identified as one cause of lower sex ratios.[44] A 2000 study of over six thousand pregnant women found that those who followed a vegetarian diet had a considerably lower sex ratio when compared to those who followed an omnivorous diet and were 23 percent less likely to give birth to a boy.[45] Could this indicate that vegetarian diets during pregnancy don't supply adequate nutrition? The low birth ratio of vegetarian women may be an indication of physical stress caused by this eating pattern and threaten fetus viability. There is neither mention of this study, nor of the risk of spontaneous abortion of male fetuses, in the AND 2016 position statement referenced earlier.

It's tough to say; there have obviously been many studies conducted on adult vegetarians and vegans, but there's much less evidence about animal-free diets for kids.[46] It's estimated that approximately five hundred thousand children under the age of five are vegan in the US alone. Many will say that a typical Western diet, full of junk food, is also unhealthy, but there's a huge difference between a diet that includes junk food and a diet that makes it difficult to get adequate amounts of key nutrients. We just don't see a reasonable argument for limiting nutrient-dense foods in children. We're not alone in our position. While the American and British dietetic organizations maintain a vegan diet is safe for all life stages, both Germany and Switzerland specifically don't recommend vegan diets for pregnant or lactating women, infants, children, or adolescents. And in May 2019 a group of doctors from the Belgian Royal Academy of Medicine put forward a proposal to make feeding babies a vegan diet illegal. The committee stated that a vegan diet is unsuitable for unborn children, children, and adolescents, as well as pregnant and lactating women, and that feeding this population a vegan diet, which requires supplements and special medical checkups, "raises important bioethical issues." Furthermore, their position is that a vegan diet induces serious deficiencies, including low protein, vitamin B12, vitamin D, calcium, iron, zinc, iodine, DHA, and especially B12.[47]

While making certain diets "illegal" may not be a preferred course of action in the US, we think that steps should be taken to require vegan parents to sign off that they realize this diet poses serious risks, and that they are responsible for getting dietary education, taking supplements, and making mandatory frequent visits to medical and dietetic experts to monitor for signs of malnutrition and failure to thrive.

If you think that this position sounds extreme, consider the very real danger of parents who don't have the knowledge or resources they need to keep their kids healthy without animal products. To list just a few examples, in 2007 a vegan couple in Atlanta were sentenced to life in prison for the death of their malnourished six-week-old baby boy, who had been fed soy milk and apple juice.[48] This is obviously an extremely poor diet for an infant, and most parents *should* know that soy milk and juice aren't nutritional equivalents to milk or formula; however, it seems clear the couple's vegan diet informed their decision about what to give their baby. Similarly, in 2017 a Belgian court found parents guilty of inadvertently causing their seven-month-old's death after feeding him a diet of vegetable-based milks.[49] In July 2016 an Italian baby who had been raised on a vegan diet without proper supplementation was hospitalized for severe malnutrition. The fourteen-month-old boy weighed slightly more than a typical three-month-old, and in the end he was taken away from his parents.[50]

Academic journals have also published case studies looking at nutrient deficiency in the babies of breastfeeding vegan mothers. For example, a Danish article from 2009 reported severe vitamin B12 deficiency in two infants who had been breastfed by vegans.[51] A French article from the same year looked at an infant with severe deficiencies in vitamins B12, K, and D; his mother had the same deficiencies. The study authors noted, "This case highlights that a vegan diet during pregnancy followed by exclusive breast-feeding can induce nutritional deficiencies in the newborn, with clinical consequences."[52] In 2014 the *Chilean Journal of Pediatrics* presented a case report about the one-year-old daughter of a long-term vegetarian woman. The child had severe vitamin B12 deficiency that led to neurological and hematological impairment.[53]

The examples we've just pointed to are alarming, and there are more. Critics will maintain that in all these cases kids were harmed not because of a vegan diet per se but because of restricted diets lacking proper supplementation. But we think that's precisely the point. If fed a balanced diet that includes meat, dairy, and eggs, most healthy kids wouldn't need additional supplementation of these crucial nutrients. Because of case studies like this, one pediatrician has even recommended that all children with failure to thrive and certain neurological signs related to B12 deficiency be assessed for vegan diets.[54]

There just doesn't seem to be great evidence that eliminating meat is ideal for kids. To date, there has only been one controlled study that examines the effect of eating meat versus limiting meat in kids. In a 2014 study researchers evaluated the impact of the addition of meat, milk, or just additional calories to the diet of largely vegetarian children in Kenya and compared them to a control group, who received no additional food. The results were fascinating. When measured for growth, intellectual ability, behavior, and academic performance, after two years the meat group had the best outcomes by far. The milk group showed the least improvement on Raven's Progressive Matrices—a measure of fluid intelligence—even when compared to the children that didn't receive any additional calories. The meat group showed remarkably more physical ability, leadership, and physical growth during the study period. Those who only received the milk substitute lagged behind the meat group in *every* aspect. The researchers believe that these results may be related to the impact milk has on iron absorption, which influences cognitive ability. They also suggest that the improvements in performance in the meat group could be due to the intake of high-quality protein, vitamin B12, zinc, and iron in the children's diet, all of which have a positive impact on development.[55] Although this is only one study with some limitations, it's the *only* controlled study on meat in children, and basically, it suggests milk can't replace meat.

A French study looking at the safety of vegan diets in children notes,

> The vegan diet ... raises questions about its benefits for a
> growing child: adequate caloric and protein intake, quality of

essential amino acids, presence of essential fatty acids, inhibition of absorption of trace elements (including iodine, iron and zinc) and supply of various vitamins. Whereas vegan food is vitamin B12 deprived, the biggest challenge remains the vitamin B12 substitution in pregnant women, breastfeeding mothers and children at any age. Specific management by pediatricians using dietetic support and blood analyzes are required for children under vegan diet with respect of moral and ethical values related to this lifestyle choice.[56]

The Academy of Nutrition and Dietetics seems to minimize the impact of missing nutrients and the evidence pointing to how it may affect the growth and development of children following vegetarian diets. It's completely reasonable to question how the AND can definitively say that removing meat is a good idea for kids.

BOTTOM LINE: MEAT IS GOOD FOR YOU, AND DIETS THAT EXCLUDE ANIMAL PRODUCTS ARE RISKY

We hope by now you can see that criticisms of red meat are not based on strong science and that the real culprit for the growing health issues we're facing are hyperpalatable, ultraprocessed modern foods. Animal products play a critical role in a healthy omnivore diet, and those who eliminate all animal products can face serious health problems. It can be a huge challenge to get the protein and other nutrients we need to thrive without animal products, especially without overconsuming calories and adding countless supplements. Overwhelmingly, the evidence shows that the optimal human diet contains animal products.

To recap, we've laid out for you some of the reasons why meat is unfairly maligned from a nutritional perspective. The studies condemning meat are based on observational research and food frequency questionnaires, which are full of bias and flawed methodology. Observational research can only show associations, not prove causation. Studies that have adjusted for confounding factors (smoking, drinking, and other lifestyle factors) have shown no difference in mortality between those who eat meat and those who don't. We've also explained the critical importance of protein, how it can make people feel full for fewer calories and more micronutrients than plant-based sources like beans and rice. There's also some pretty compelling evidence that, indeed, humans are omnivores, we have been eating animal products for a very long time, and animal protein and fats contain many of the critical components we need to thrive. Those who eliminate meat from their diets, especially pregnant women and young children, are putting themselves at risk for nutrient deficiencies, some of which could even lead to permanent brain damage if there's no intervention.

All right, then, you might say. Even if meat isn't bad for my health, raising cattle for food is still environmentally irresponsible and ethically questionable, right? While we don't see a huge *nutrition* benefit to choosing grass-finished beef over typical beef, there are certainly very good reasons to choose cattle managed and handled well. In part two we'll explain why the environmental case against beef is unfair. We'll then move to the ethical reason why eliminating animals from our food system could cause more harm than good, and finally, address specific actions you can take to improve your health while eating a diet that is both sustainable and ethical.

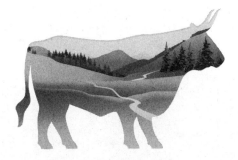

PART II

THE ENVIRONMENTAL CASE FOR (BETTER) MEAT

CHAPTER 7

WHAT ROLE DOES LIVESTOCK PLAY IN OUR ENVIRONMENT?

Although it is perhaps a painful reality, human nature doesn't lend itself well to looking at long-term solutions. In his book *Collapse*, the anthropologist and historian Jared Diamond writes:

> Consider a narrow river valley below a high dam, such that if the dam burst, the resulting flood of water would drown people for a considerable distance downstream. When attitude pollsters ask people downstream of the dam how concerned they are about the dam bursting, it's not surprising that fear of a dam burst is lowest far downstream and increases among residents increasingly close to the dam. Surprisingly, though, after you get just a few miles below the dam, where fear of the dam bursting is found to be highest, concern then falls off to zero as you approach closer to the dam! That is, the people living immediately under the dam, the ones most certain to be drowned in a dam burst, profess unconcern. That's because of psychological denial: the only way of

preserving one's sanity while looking up every day at the dam is to deny the possibility that it could burst.

One could argue that similar psychological denialism exists today around the topic of the environment. Some people do not care about the environment because "that's a problem for another day." Others care deeply but their proposed solutions, although well meaning, are largely divorced from reality, cost (both economic and social), and efficacy (will the proposed interventions to "save the world" make things better, or worse?). We have already pointed to a fair number of historical precedents of good intentions paving a path, if not to hell, to a place no one wanted to go (decisions made around what constitutes a "healthy" diet has likely not only made people less healthy but has accelerated and entrenched perhaps the most injurious elements of our food production system, for both human and global health). We feel that the current argument that cattle are one of the main contributors to our climate crisis is yet another such example; though we should all share the goal of caring for the environment, we'll now walk you through why a world without livestock is not necessarily any better off.

THE ROLE OF ANIMALS IN OUR ENVIRONMENT

Life on earth is complex. It may be a bit counterintuitive, but certain systems, particularly those that involve shifting both energy and resources (such as economies, ecosystems, and growing children), not only benefit from but thrive upon complexity. In physics, the term for this is resiliency, while the noted author Nassim Taleb coined the term "antifragile."

Whatever term we use, it is important to understand the difference between things like economies, ecosystems, and living things and things like internal combustion engines, computers, and chandeliers. The former are made stronger and arguably healthier with some degree of stress and challenge (not too much, but not too little), whereas the latter tend to malfunction or simply break when subjected to stress. This may seem inconsequential, but missing this distinction could lead to well-intentioned but disastrous activity.

For example, a grassland, and all the multitude of plants and animals that call it home, can be damaged by either too much or too little stress. What do we mean by that? A grassland may be damaged by improper grazing, which might lead environmental groups to seek political interventions preventing future grazing. For a brief time the grassland may benefit while the pressure of overgrazing is removed, but over the long term it will suffer because its ecosystem evolved with plants *and* animals. The right solution here might not be all or nothing. Rather, we might have to start looking at how natural systems work and doing our best to support those processes instead of circumventing them.

GRASSWORLD

Perhaps one of the best ways to appreciate the power and importance of environmental complexity is to imagine building a world from scratch and consider how diversity affects the relative health and vitality of this planet.

Imagine, for a moment, a near-future science fiction story in which astronomers, sequestered in their tech-heavy observatories, make a startling discovery: a planet, the same size as the Earth, is on a collision course with our solar system. Initially, pandemonium ensues; nine months later, birth rates soar, as it appears this may literally be the end of the world. But one astronomer and mathematician carefully assesses the data and makes a remarkable prediction. The new world will enter the inner solar system and take up a permanent orbit on the far side of the sun, exactly opposite the Earth, in what is called the third Lagrangian point. Pandemonium and birth rates spike yet again, as not only is our world unlikely to end but it appears our new celestial neighbor is a near-perfect replica of our own modest abode. This new world has mountains, oceans, lakes, and rivers. It has shifting weather patterns, including tornadoes and hurricanes. It has an identical mix of minerals in the crust and gases in the atmosphere as the Earth. Indeed, the only thing our new neighbor lacks is *life*. The planet is absolutely, completely sterile.

The opportunity is astounding: a whole new world. Some suggest we should send missions to mine its mineral resources and bring these back to Earth. Others, with perhaps a bit more forethought (and understanding of how much energy space flight really entails) suggest we terraform the planet and transform the lifeless sphere into a new home. This suggestion is met with great zeal, but the process quickly grinds to a halt as the debate begins on how to actually *do* this. Where to start? Trees? Water lilies? Some insightful people suggest the most banal of vegetative options: grass. The proposal is met with equal parts strident protest and enthusiastic acceptance. On the one hand, people accuse big corporations of wanting to convert the whole planet into a golf course, but others recognize the wisdom of this plan. Nearly 40 percent of the earth's surface is grassland. Many warm season grasses are C_4 plants, which makes them grow much faster than cool season grasses and trees, which are C_3 plants. The evolution of C_4 plants in recent geological history was indeed responsible for allowing grasses to conquer the continental interiors that previously struggled with much life. That's because they can grow faster while giving up less water and consequently continue growth at warmer temperatures.

Grass it is! A three-thousand-acre test area is picked and an unmanned spacecraft overflies the area at the beginning of what would be spring on the new world, sprinkling seeds from a low altitude. Light rains, cool mornings, and warm afternoons provide the perfect environment for the grass to sprout and take hold.

Unfortunately, satellite images of the area paint a bleak picture: the hearty grass seeds have sprouted but quickly died. What went wrong? In assessing the initial plan, a vocal group that advocated for sending enormous quantities of dung into space had been dismissed as crackpots. But it appears they were onto something. Although we are well acquainted with the portion of grasslands above the surface, below ground an intricate web exists in which roots, microbes, and fungi work synergistically to capture energy from the sun and mine minerals from the soil. This work is performed via a remarkable symbiosis amongst the various microorganisms, which are ultimately fed by the plants. In short, without animal dung, the microbes were absent.

A second attempt is made, sending microbes and dung with the grass seeds.

Things progress much better this time, but after a few months the whole system collapses again. Some of the soil organisms can fix atmospheric nitrogen, but after time the grass appears to have finally run out. Also, the only places plants could grow were low-lying areas. Even a light rain appeared to wash nutrients downhill, leaving hillsides barren and prone to erosion. The grass itself seemed oddly stunted upon second-generation germination, as though the seeds needed "help."

Consultation with more experts elicits the suggestion to send grazing animals, such as cattle, to this new world. Cattle manure has proven a vital component in healthy grassland ecosystems. Instead of flying vast sums of dung across the inner solar system, why not deposit "factories" that can make effectively unlimited quantities? The cows move around, breaking up the soil, but also moving nutrients (and grass seeds) to higher elevations via dung and urine. Their impact also stimulates new root growth and increases the biology of the soil.

Things *really* take off with this third attempt. Not only does the grass thrive—it expands beyond the intended boundaries of the test area. The cows breached the safety fencing and did what cows do: pee and poo.

And eat.

And move.

And breed.

The grass expands beyond the wildest dreams of the scientists, but to their shock and horror, the cow population outstrips the expanding grasslands.

It takes a few years, but eventually the cattle destroy the grasslands, and their population plummets. Our neighbor in the solar system is once again a largely sterile, lifeless world. But the promise of a new world is too great to give up; what appears to be needed is a means of controlling the cow population.

So a fourth mission sends microbes, dung, grass seeds, cows—and, eventually, wolves. Things develop just as they did in the third attempt, but this time, after the grasslands have begun expanding and the cattle population has grown, a population of wolves are introduced to the planet. Things work. A dynamic equilibrium is found. The grassland slowly spreads around the planet, supported by the activity of the cows, whose population is kept in check by the wolves.

The good times are short-lived, however. A few farsighted scientists point out that the system is remarkably fragile and only one catastrophe away from complete collapse. What if one of the bacteria mutates and attacks the wolves? Or one of the molds takes over the grass? Or a virus could wipe out the whole herd of cattle. Just one of these three species dies, and the entire system goes with it. The whole new planet is one pandemic away from yet again being as lifeless as Mars.

The solution? As quickly as possible, introduce as many new species of plants, animals, bacteria, and fungi to increase the biodiversity and thereby stabilize the planetary ecology. Introduce rainforest plants and animals in wet, warm areas; introduce drought-adapted critters to areas likely to be desert. Add penguins, polar bears, lichen, and seals at the poles. Make sure to get some algae, seaweed, and a host of animals in the oceans. Once the basic spark of life has been established, work to provide as much diversity of plants, animals, bacteria, and fungi as possible.

COMPLEXITY ENSURES RESILIENCE

According to *Merriam-Webster's Collegiate Dictionary*, an ecosystem is "the complex of a community of organisms and its environment functioning as an ecological unit." The key word here is *complex*. Recalling the lesson from our Grassworld experiment above, it's clear that the more diverse and complex an ecosystem is, the healthier and more resilient it is. This is true all over the world.

BACK TO EARTH: HOW CATTLE AND OTHER GRAZERS CAN BENEFIT LAND

Deserts and arctic regions are considered fragile because of their relative lack of diversity. Hillsides need inputs from animals that carry nutrients up from the fertile valleys through their manure. Without these animals and their dung, which helps to grow vegetation, which locks the soil in place and slows the passage of water down the hillside (and actually encourages the seeping of surface water into groundwater), we're much more susceptible to landslides.

How did North America develop such a fertile breadbasket? It wasn't because farmers were growing wheat or tomatoes for thousands of years; it was because millions of bison and other ruminants were grazing and fertilizing the soil, driving the solar-fueled process that typifies grasslands. Without ruminants chomping, grass just grows, oxidizes (this is a slow, nonproductive process in which sunlight slowly turns organic matter into the biological equivalent of ashtray leavings), and eventually dies. When ruminants have to move (whether because a predator is after them or because a farmer guides them into a new area with electric fencing), they only eat the top portion of the plants, which maintains the root mass and prevents overgrazing. Perennial grasses (grasses that come back year after year), common in grasslands, have deeper root systems and are often part of a latent seed bank (seeds of plants that have been lying around dormant waiting for favorable conditions to reemerge and grow). Ruminant manure inoculates the soil with beneficial nutrients and microbes, increasing the biodiversity underground and leading to a much more resilient soil profile. The urine and manure from animals increase moisture to the soil and the microbial diversity of bacteria and fungi that form "the gut" for the soil in a symbiotic system. Grasslands need ruminants to be healthy.

The carbon sequestration process starts when the grasses, legumes, and forbs go through photosynthesis. The leaves of these plants take carbon dioxide out of the air and convert that CO_2 to oxygen. The plants also exude carbon down through their roots to feed the microbes. This carbon, which is essentially sugar, is known as exudate. Various soil microbes exchange sugar for nutrients like minerals, which the plants need to grow via the root system (known as the rhizosphere). Fungal networks connected to this root system form pathways for the microbes to move through the soil. These fungal networks also produce acids that break down minerals that make the minerals bioavailable to the plants. Minerals have to be made bioavailable for the plants to be able to use them. The increased carbon in the ground changes the structure of the soil, providing more open spaces—kind of like a sponge. Thus, healthy soil is less compact, and can absorb significantly more rainwater than brittle, compacted, plowed, or overgrazed land.

Over 90 percent of the pasture's health lies underground. Continuous grazing, where the land is not allowed to rest, depletes the root biomass, increases the bare ground, lowers soil organic carbon reserves, and contributes to soil erosion and compaction, decreasing its water-holding capacity. Exposed soils—which can result from overgrazing, overstocking, or poor cropping—emit greenhouse gases. These practices also send organic matter sediments into waterways. Areas like the anoxic dead zone of the Gulf of Mexico, as well as the declining numbers of North American pollinators, are examples of what can happen from soil erosion.

As we mentioned earlier in our Grassworld scenario, animals can bring nutrients up hills, something that is otherwise difficult to do without tractors and chemicals. In the wild, ruminants graze in the meadows but then go uphill to avoid predators, and when they do, they bring with them fermented nutrients (in the form of manure) to the hillsides. Rain washes it down, which is why valleys are fertile. If we completely eliminated ruminants, hillsides would no longer have the nutrients they need, we'd see more landslides from soil degradation, and valleys would no longer be as fertile as they once were.

There are many creative uses for grazing animals that are yet to be fully explored, like "silvopasture," or combining trees, pasture, and grazers in a mutually beneficial way; the trees provide shelter for the grazers, the pasture provides them food, and the animals, in turn, provide fertilizer for the plants. In such a system, cattle might be incorporated through coconut trees in the tropics or in apple orchards in the United States. Farmers can also use "pasture cropping." In this method, farmers plant cover crops (crops that are grown to protect and enrich the soil) in their fields to control weeds and reduce the need for synthetic nitrogen. Rather than using herbicides to burn down these cover crops in no-till systems, farmers can use ruminants to graze down the cover crops, after which the cash crops can be planted. At the end of the cash crop season, farmers can then also allow animals to graze crop residues where vegetables and grains have been previously harvested. Many corn and wheat farmers allow cattle grazing on their fields after the harvest (something that's not well accounted for in land-use studies—which will become relevant soon). These mixed agricultural models offer interesting opportunities for increasing fertility of the soil while also increasing the yield per acre of the land. If you can produce both apples *and* beef from an orchard, bringing in cattle to manage the grass instead of mowing, it's a win-win. If grazing animals can increase biodiversity, both underground and above, then a field of well-managed cattle could certainly be better for the earth than a gigantic plowed field of soy sprayed with chemicals.

HAVE WE MISTAKENLY RE-CREATED GRASSWORLD?

Via our modern agriculture practices, we have, through good intentions, but unfortunate misunderstanding, constructed a food system that is dangerously close to the earliest iteration of Grassworld—wiping out all other life that once inhabited that land to make room for just one single crop. All the birds, frogs, rabbits, and other life that once lived there is eliminated. We need lots of chemical inputs to fertilize the soil because there's no animal manure to do so. We also need tons of chemical pesticides and fungicides to kill what will want to take over this crop. In the process, we kill more insects and birds, we destroy the soil, these chemicals run off into rivers, killing fish and the animals that depend on the fish. Industrial monocropping, though it can temporarily feed a lot of people some cheap calories, is a horror show to nature. Growing food is a biological process, but we've taken this biological process and turned it into a chemical one. Not only is this system more precarious than we'd like, the very processes supporting industrial agriculture are literally blowing the soil from beneath our feet.

By trucking in and applying synthetic nitrogen and key nutrients such as phosphorus, we have been able to drive food production forward, but it comes at a cost: we are losing our topsoil and the tiny but vitally important life within it.

Just how much life is left in our topsoil is a matter of debate. In 2014 Maria Helena Semedo, an economist and deputy general director of climate and natural resources at the Food and Agriculture Organization, estimated that we have only about *sixty years* of farming left at our current rate of topsoil degradation before the soil is untenable for future food production. A sobering estimate.

Although this "sixty harvests" number sounds like a convincing statistic, when we looked for the root science on this topic . . . there was none. It might be tempting to use the Malthusian prediction to cement our position, but the number appears to have been related off the cuff at a conference. And yet it's become so entrenched in the climate zeitgeist that even asking for source material can get one into trouble as a "denier." Even so, we asked, and the information to support the claim was not just lacking—it simply does not exist.

Now, a bit of context is in order. Reasonable analysis of the global status of soil health paints a sobering picture: many locations are categorized as "poor," a few as "moderate," and one can find the occasional unicorn that could be called "healthy." The anemic state of our soils *is* a problem, as it requires intensification of synthetic fertilizers, pesticides, herbicides, and so on, while also minimizing water retention, nutrient content, and a host of other features that are important for a food system that will last us as long as our species would like to exist. So, yes, regenerative practices, which includes the proper use of animals, are critical to a sustainable future. Although the precise dating may be dubious, the process of our soils declining under the current system is both accurate and critical to properly address. Continuing our current farming practices, growing more and more plants (as Planet of the Monocrops, let's face it, is nothing but row crops built by the industrial food system), will not solve this problem.

As we mentioned in the introduction, this is a remarkably complex topic and one that requires more than a fifteen-second sound bite to begin to unpack. Although it's laudable when celebrities bring their substantial influence to an agenda, it's important to focus that energy in a way that improves the problem.

Leonardo DiCaprio's recent documentary *Before the Flood* raises awareness of how important it is that we make changes to avoid environmental ruin. This is great, and the film is powerful. Unfortunately, DiCaprio makes a titanic mistake when he stands next to climatology professor Gidon Eshel as he recommends eating less beef and more chicken to help the environment.

On the surface, this may seem like a great idea: chickens are small, and cows are big. It's got to be a "win" to shift our eating this way, right? Unfortunately, Eshel has a very shallow understanding of the topic. Let's take a look.

Again, animals like chickens play an important albeit underappreciated role in natural food systems. Generally, large numbers of grazing animals produce prodigious amounts of dung, which is an incubator for a host of insects, worms, and other unseemly critters. The ecological niche of birds like chickens is to play "clean up," eating insects, larvae, and worms in close proximity to ruminant dung. If you have ever owned chickens, you will appreciate they make their own constant contributions to the nitrogen cycle. Although some egg cartons and advertising trumpets "vegetarian-fed chickens," chickens are not grazing animals. They are opportunistic omnivores that operate more like miniature velociraptors than grazers. Chickens can and will eat just about anything, including small amounts of grass, but they must also have worms, bugs, small rodents, and seasonal seed pods of plants such as grasses and grains. As monogastric animals, chickens have a very different digestive system from ruminants like cows, which have a complex digestive system that can break down the cellulosic material of plants, turning inaccessible (for humans and many animals) plant matter into food.

What is the takeaway to all this? In our modern industrial food system, cows eat mainly grass. There is a widely held belief that cattle consume large amounts of grain and that this is effectively "taking food away" from what could otherwise feed humans, but this is incorrect. We'll look at this topic in depth later in the book, but for now, we want to clarify: the vast majority of food eaten by cattle comes from grass, and the grains that are fed to cattle are mainly the remnants of ethanol production and the leftover "straw" from grain harvest. Chickens, by contrast, are almost exclusively fed on grain and soybean meal. Our modern food system is so good at providing for us that these quirks and nuances are easy to overlook, but it was not so long ago that chicken was a treat consumed only occasionally. The saying "A chicken in every pot" has been erroneously attributed to 1928 presidential candidate Herbert Hoover. In fact, a group of supporters of Hoover's political campaign coined this phrase, but the promise was alluring: before the intensification of our food system, there was not extra grain available to raise chickens en masse as is common practice today. The bulk of animal products consumed came from grazing animals, for reasons that are hopefully becoming clearer. Eating chicken today is inextricably linked with modern industrial farming practices that are unsustainable in the long term.

Despite millions of dollars invested in the project and backing from the National Geographic Society, no one involved in Mr. DiCaprio's film seems to have bothered to confirm if the "more chicken, less beef" recommendation actually made good environmental sense. Or perhaps someone did ask these questions, but those inconvenient truths were abandoned on the cutting room floor.

GROWING FOOD TAKES ENERGY

Whatever shortcomings our hypothetical Grassworld may have with regards to diversity, it is a process that could, in theory, go on and on. For how long? Well, at the base of Grassworld's ecosystem is grass, which relies on photosynthesis (and manure) to grow. Barring other planetary catastrophes, this type of system *could* go on until the Sun shifts from hydrogen to helium fusion, becoming a red giant and possibly engulfing the earth in five billion years. This is a good bit longer than life has existed on earth thus far, and the process is effectively "free." So long as sunlight falls upon the earth, this story could continue. Part of the case we will make is that we should look to ways to maximize this process of energy capture via photosynthesis while also protecting (even expanding) biodiversity. The more diverse life is, the more likely life is to continue, particularly if this life is tied to an energy source that is, if not infinite, at least likely to last "a very long time."

CHAPTER 8

CAN A SUSTAINABLE FOOD SYSTEM EXIST WITHOUT ANIMALS?

In the previous chapter, we wanted to provide a framework for understanding the role of animals in the environment and a means of critically assessing the competing ideologies surrounding sustainability. As you read on, we will ask you to consider the following points to help you assess whether a given recommendation or criticism of a food system has merit.

1. If climate change is of concern (and it should be), interventions should reduce net greenhouse gas levels. If possible, the intervention should even present an option for reversing this process.

2. As much as possible, the energy needed to raise our food should come from the sun, not fossil fuel inputs, and our methods should support complex, resilient ecosystems. The

exact methods used will have to change around the world—
it should come as no surprise that a solution suited to the
Mongolian steppe is likely to look different from one suited
to the interior of the Amazon—but interventions should be
critically assessed with the criterion of energy inputs versus
outputs in mind.

3. Recommended dietary practices and food production
   methods must consider the limited window humanity has with
   regards to topsoil. There is little debate that should topsoil
   largely disappear, so shall we.

4. While we are considering biodiversity, it behooves us to also
   value cultural diversity. The current monocrop industrial food
   process has effectively crushed traditional food systems,
   replacing them both at the production and consumption levels
   with what is arguably a less diverse, less nutritious diet. Is
   it reasonable for a few wealthy, largely white vegan-centric
   activists to push a global food agenda that would make
   verboten every other food system on the planet?

The second point is salient. The bulk of modern life, including food
production, is driven by the use of fossil fuels. It is conceivable that
energy sources such as solar or nuclear could make energy so abundant that the industrial food system could continue while largely
ceasing to produce carbon dioxide. While this development is something to be hoped for, it will not solve the issue raised in the third
point: the looming threat of topsoil loss.

Whether in political talking points or ecological systems, diversity is a laudable and important concept. Knowing as we do that
diversity is invaluable to ecosystems, how can anyone seriously propose that it's in our best interests to stop raising and eating animals
and instead cover every inch of farmable land with the same three
crops? This would continue the trend of the past sixty years, with
wheat, rice, and corn taking center stage in the diets of most people. Modern agricultural practices have allowed us to dramatically

increase our numbers to the point where humans have expanded to nearly every corner of the globe. But in this process we have inadvertently shifted what was once a highly diversified planetary ecosystem into something much closer to Grassworld.

A move that seems clearly at odds with a long-term sustainable and resilient future is decreasing the net biodiversity of the planet by shifting the bulk of calories consumed to a few cereal crops. The widespread use of synthetic fertilizers, pesticides, herbicides, and soil tillage that this approach entails has disastrous ramifications to plant, animal, insect, and microbial populations. Plowing the soil disturbs the connective "glue" that holds it together and also releases carbon into the atmosphere. As mentioned earlier, the current system is highly productive—for now. But topsoil degradation makes future harvests uncertain at best (this fact is part of what drives the fervor for hydroponics, which as we will see offers little in the way of regenerating soil health.) Although difficult to predict, it is reasonable to assume that as topsoil degrades, harvests may be negatively affected, which generally involves a "doubling down" on things like synthetic fertilizer, which may accelerate this process.

Modern food production is highly energy intensive, and the bulk of this energy is currently supplied by fossil fuels. The Haber-Bosch process converts atmospheric nitrogen (largely unusable by most plants other than legumes) into ammonia. The ammonia can then be used as a robust nitrogen source for crops. But this miracle of the Green Revolution of the twentieth century actually appears to exacerbate soil degradation. Synthetic fertilizers bypass the complex natural processes established over millennia involving sunlight, plants, animals, and a host of soil microbes.

It's difficult to find voices in science or even the media that advocate for the elimination of species (with the possible exception of some camps that think the removal of Homo sapiens would be, on the whole, a good thing) so we can agree that activities that foster biodiversity are likely a good thing. Additionally, if we are to be concerned about greenhouse gas emissions, it makes sense to find solutions that minimize the need for inputs like synthetic fertilizer. If *that* all holds water (both analogy and property of healthy soil . . .), one must wonder how a row-crop-centric food system, which hinges on the use of these unsustainable inputs, can be put forward as a solution to global food security.

WHAT ABOUT LAB MEAT AND HYDROPONICS?

Some starry-eyed optimists have suggested novel ideas such as lab-grown meat and hydroponics as a solution to global food needs. They've been presented as both sustainable and more ethical than natural, biological agriculture practices. Neither process improves the soil nor takes advantage of the sun as a free energy source. The lab-grown meat idea, in particular, has been the darling of Silicon Valley tech types; hundreds of millions of dollars of venture capital has flowed into these projects.

Shelving the ethics discussion for the next part of this book, the sustainability claim is fascinating on many levels: raising meat of any variety requires a significant energetic input. In the case of ruminants on grassland, as we saw in the last chapter, the energy is supplied by the sun, and we achieve a host of knock-on benefits such as carbon sequestration, soil water retention, maintenance of ecosystems, and, critically, topsoil production. In the case of lab-grown meat, we must either build a lab (an enormous energy investment, and whenever we say "energy investment," you can usually take that to be synonymous with "greenhouse gas emissions") or, more ideally, take over space that can be repurposed. OK, a light industrial space is outfitted to begin growing lab meat. Muscle cells taken from an animal (typically a cow fetus) are placed in a growth medium, kept sterile, not too hot, nor too cold, and over time the cells grow into what is effectively "meat."

In a 2015 paper titled "Anticipatory Life Cycle Analysis of In Vitro Biomass Cultivation for Cultured Meat Production in the United States," researchers looked at the land use and other resources that would be required to produce cultured meat in labs.[1] Here are the steps involved in producing it:

First, soybeans and corn are grown and processed to produce peptides and starch for the process. Vitamins and minerals are also required, which must be mined, isolated, and processed. After some initial production of glucose (from the corn) into amino acids and basal media, these raw ingredients are then transported along with the animal-derived cells to the facility. Growth factors—that is, animal sera—that are currently required for the process were not calculated into the study. (It should be noted that the industry is currently developing serum-free media (SFM) out of soy hydrolysate, and the study authors anticipated cultured meat would be produced in an SFM; however, as of the writing of this book, this is not the current practice. What's more, the extractive agricultural methods of soy production should leave one questioning if this is really a giant leap forward in terms of environmental sustainability.)

A large bioreactor is filled with "basal medium," which for this study they assumed would be soy, but could be another crop. Ammonia builds up and has to be released. "Donated" cells from animals multiply for the first seventy-two hours, then a mixture of glucose, oxygen, and glutamine is added for further duplication of cells. Interestingly, the fact that this is made from baby cow biopsies doesn't sit well with vegans, and from what we've read, they do not consider lab meat to be vegan approved.

Soy hydrolysate concentration is added, and the mixture gives off alanine, ammonia, and lactate. The mixture then grows on a "scaffold" mimicking the structure of animal tissue. Energy is required for climate control, lighting, and to run the bioreactor, which mixes, aerates, and regulates the temperature of the culture. The growing tissue is quite susceptible to contamination. The tanks must be rinsed and sanitized after each batch with deionized water and sodium hydroxide. The process requires 74,600 liters of water to yield 555 kilograms of biomass.

At the end of the day, the energy required for the process far exceeds any type of current livestock production model. In this paper, they found that the land use required for the inputs exceeded that anticipated in a previous study by twenty times. Additionally, the global warming potential (GWP) of lab meat far exceeds pork or poultry production. The report claims lab meat is better than the GWP of beef; however, as we'll explain in chapter nine, cattle's biogenic greenhouse gases are part of a cycle and are not a fair comparison to the emissions created from fossil fuels.

What's more, the row crops grown for this process, if not grown differently, destroy the topsoil. Ironically, if we were to try to produce the grain inputs for lab meat in a regenerative way, we'd need to use ruminant animals to do this—sort of defeating the purpose of nonanimal meat!

A quick note on hydroponics: this is the process of growing plants in liquid, sand, or gravel, without soil. Use of hydroponics in certain locations could offer a degree of variety that would be tough to achieve naturally (like hydroponically growing fresh greens in Iceland, for example, which is largely run by renewable geothermal energy). Hydroponics have been highly (wink, wink) effective for marijuana production and growing lettuce—a plant that's effectively crunchy water, nutritionally speaking—and little else. One does *not* grow corn, soy, rice, or other foods in any appreciable amounts via this process.

When a life cycle analysis is performed on things like lab-grown meat and hydroponic vegetables, it's clear that these systems generally require enormous amounts of energy to produce any appreciable quantity of food, and, again, at present, most of this energy is coming from fossil fuel sources. Advocates that portray lab meat and hydroponics as a viable option to feed the world have failed to do some simple, albeit boring, arithmetic.

So why this huge interest in lab meats? Certainly, there are some smart people in Silicon Valley that must have done similar calculations, right?

The real benefit in lab meat is the fact that it's a highly technologically driven food. As Sarah Martin, assistant professor with the Department of Political Science at Memorial University of

Newfoundland, pointed out at the Future of Protein conference at the University of Ottawa, to grow lab meat you need cell lines, cell culture media, scaffolding and structuring, and bioreactors—all these things that can be patented. If the lab-meat folks can get the public to accept it as an alternative to meat, then they will own the lucrative intellectual property license on this technique. There's not a ton of profit to be made in animal agriculture, but there's gobs of money to be made in processing foods into something new. If they can control the whole supply chain and make a product that few others can make, which they'll convince the public is better for the environment and causes less harm to animals, the profit margins on a product like this are enormous. No longer will they have to deal with people buying meat directly from the farmer up the street—it can all come from the lab. This side of the meat production story is not dissimilar to what has happened with various crops: patentable seeds are foisted on farmers, who lose the ability to bank their own seeds. Where once there was independence, there is now serfdom.

Is lab meat going to build topsoil and increase biodiversity? Will producing meat from more synthetic chemical–produced mono-crops really cause less harm to our planet and to all of the animals who need habitat? What is the goal of our time here? Is it support-ing intellectual property held by a few multinational corporations, or can we try to build a resilient food system that relies more on solar power (photosynthesis) and less on fossil fuels? If the goal is to build a resilient ecosystem, how can we do this?

CHAPTER 9

ARE CATTLE CONTRIBUTING TO CLIMATE CHANGE?

You've heard it time and time again: cow farts are ruining our planet! (Perhaps a pedantic bit of hairsplitting, but cattle don't really fart methane; they mostly belch it as a part of their digestive process.) We're often told by mainstream media that livestock are worse than all transportation when it comes to greenhouse gases and climate change. However, please allow us to explain why this is misleading and actually not accurate.

These are the three main greenhouse gases (GHG) associated with agriculture:

- carbon dioxide (CO_2), primarily released in plowing, cutting trees, and when burning fossil fuels
- methane (CH_4), which comes mostly from rice and belching cattle
- nitrous oxide (N_2O), largely coming from the application of fertilizers

Each of these can be measured in terms of its greenhouse warming potential (GWP), a quantification of how much heat a GHG traps in the atmosphere. It compares the amount of heat a particular gas would trap to the amount a similar mass of carbon dioxide would trap. So, carbon dioxide accordingly has a GWP of 1; methane has a GWP of 28–36; and nitrous oxide comes in at 265–298. However, according to the EPA, each of these gases remains in the atmosphere for a different amount of time. Carbon dioxide remains active for thousands of years, methane only lasts about ten, and nitrous oxide about one hundred.[1] It is perhaps also worth mentioning that when we talk about carbon capture, that process is not independent of methane . . . Methane is composed of a carbon atom with four hydrogens, and it factors directly into the carbon sequestration potential of properly managed grazing animals that we will detail in this section. Both of us have received a remarkable amount of confused pushback when talking about the total carbon footprint in this story. An unfortunately typical response has been "OK, yeah, cattle can sequester carbon, but what about the methane! That's the real issue! Who is paying you guys for this misinformation?!"

We will illustrate to you that the methane claims are largely overblown, and show how well-managed cattle are actually part of the solution to climate change because their impact may actually be a net carbon sink.

WHERE DO METHANE EMISSIONS COME FROM?

Methane emissions come from anaerobic breakdown of organic materials (like your composting kitchen scraps), and in the case of food production, some from ruminant digestion. Although (as we will see) there are *many* contributors to methane production, oddly, the villains in the popular story are grazing animals. And we'd like to make the case that getting worried about methane production from *any* biological process is reductionistic (and alarmingly silly). Why? Because methane produced via biological process is part of

CATTLE CARBON CYCLING VS FOSSIL FUELS

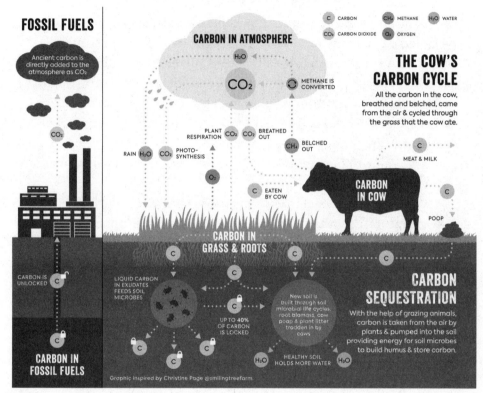

FOSSIL FUELS

Ancient carbon is directly added to the atmosphere as CO₂

CO₂

CARBON IS UNLOCKED C

CARBON IN FOSSIL FUELS

CARBON IN ATMOSPHERE

H₂O

CO₂

RAIN H₂O CO₂ PHOTO-SYNTHESIS

PLANT RESPIRATION CO₂ CO₂ BREATHED OUT

O₂

C EATEN BY COW

METHANE IS CONVERTED

CH₄ BELCHED OUT

C CARBON   CH₄ METHANE   H₂O WATER
CO₂ CARBON DIOXIDE   O₂ OXYGEN

THE COW'S CARBON CYCLE

All the carbon in the cow, breathed and belched, came from the air & cycled through the grass that the cow ate.

C

MEAT & MILK

CARBON IN COW

C

POOP

CARBON IN GRASS & ROOTS

C   C   C

LIQUID CARBON IN EXUDATES FEEDS SOIL MICROBES

UP TO **40%** OF CARBON IS LOCKED

New soil is built through soil microbial life cycles, root biomass, cow poop & plant litter trodden in by cows

C   C   H₂O   HEALTHY SOIL HOLDS MORE WATER   H₂O

CARBON SEQUESTRATION

With the help of grazing animals, carbon is taken from the air by plants & pumped into the soil providing energy for soil microbes to build humus & store carbon.

Graphic inspired by Christine Page @smilingtreefarm

a system, provides no net inputs to the system, and perhaps most important, is caused by living organisms! Let's take a closer look.

As you can see from the above illustration, inspired by Christine Page of Smiling Tree Farm in Britain, it's critical to understand that the methane emitted from cattle are part of the natural, or "biogenic," carbon cycle, whereas fossil fuels are not. Fossil fuels come from "ancient" carbon that has been locked underground for millions of years, and when it is extracted, it's adding new carbon to the atmosphere, which lasts thousands of years. In the case of cattle, they are transforming existing carbon, in the form of grass and other fibrous materials, into methane as part of their digestive process. Methane is then belched out, and after about ten years is broken back down into water and carbon dioxide molecules. The CO_2 and H_2O are cycled back to grow more grass, and the cycle continues.

Industrial animal production, with its manure lagoons, is indeed a significant source of methane, but these are largely from the pork, egg, and dairy industries. Beef feedlots generally do not use manure lagoons. And although cattle do burp methane, this is simply a natural by-product of their digestive process. Some of this breakdown and methane production would happen even if it weren't inside a bovine digestive tract. As we'll explore later, cattle are upcycling nutrients. They're converting grass and other plants that are of little nutrient value to humans into high-quality protein while improving the quality of our soil.

Concentrated animal feces from factory farms are a much different environmental issue than scattered cattle poop, urine, and hooves across grasslands in a natural system. In well-managed systems without a lot of antibiotics or drugs given to the animals, large dung beetle populations are reestablished. These dung beetles help break down manure, and recent studies found they help to mitigate methane emissions from it.[2] How do they do this? Methane is produced in low-oxygen environments. As they tunnel through manure, dung beetles provide ways for oxygen to circulate, preventing methane formation.

Let's also not forget that before the mid-1800s, there were an estimated thirty to sixty million bison, over ten million elk, thirty to forty million white-tailed deer, ten to thirteen million mule deer, and thirty-five to one hundred million pronghorn and caribou roaming North America.[3] Yet nobody seems to acknowledge this when citing current "devastating" herbivore numbers. According to a paper published in the *Journal of Animal Science*, in presettlement America, methane emissions were about 82 percent of current emissions from farmed and wild ruminants.[4]

In a 2003 report from the Food and Agriculture Organization and the International Atomic Energy Agency titled "Belching Ruminants, a Minor Player in Atmospheric Methane," researchers concluded that cattle are unfairly blamed for their methane emissions as a significant contributor to GHG emissions:

Since 1999 atmospheric methane concentrations have leveled off while the world population of ruminants has increased at an accelerated rate. Prior to 1999, world ruminant populations were increasing at the rate of 9.15 million head/year but since 1999 this rate has increased to 16.96 million head/year. Prior to 1999 there was a strong relationship between change in atmospheric methane concentrations and the world ruminant populations. However, since 1999 this strong relation has disappeared. This change in relationship between the atmosphere and ruminant numbers suggests that the role of ruminants in greenhouse gases may be less significant than originally thought, with other sources and sinks playing a larger role in global methane accounting.[5]

According to a recent NASA study, the largest contributors to methane are the fossil fuels, fires, and wetlands or rice farming. One teragram of methane weighs about the same as two hundred thousand elephants (about 1.1 million tons), and the total amount in the atmosphere is rising at a rate of approximately 25 teragrams per year. The researchers were able to find the exact cause of the recent increases in methane: "The team showed that about 17 teragrams per year of the increase is due to fossil fuels, another 12 is from wetlands or rice farming, while fires are decreasing by about 4 teragrams per year. The three numbers combine to 25 teragrams a year—the same as the observed increase."[6]

If you look into this a little more, you'll find a shockingly high percentage comes from wetland rice production: 6 to 29 percent of human-generated methane emissions[7] and 2.5 percent of overall global anthropogenic emissions.[8] (Instead of Meatless Mondays, should we call for rice-free Fridays?)

Those who might want to throw cows under the bus for producing methane should also be prepared to account for additional inputs from the natural world. A small population of shellfish in the Baltic Sea is estimated to produce as much methane as twenty thousand dairy cattle. The takeaways of many after a cursory understanding of the topic can be stark. According to researchers from

Stockholm University and Cardiff University, "These small yet very abundant animals may play an important, but so far neglected, role in regulating the emissions of greenhouse gases in the sea." An article about the team's research stated,

> To arrive at their results the team analysed trace gas, isotopes and molecules from the worms and clams, known as polychaetes and bivalves respectively, taken from ocean sediments in the Baltic Sea. The team analysed both the direct and indirect contribution that these groups were having on methane and nitrous oxide production in the sea. The results showed that sediments containing clams and worms increased methane production by a factor of eight compared to **completely bare sediments**.[9]

As a result, the study authors urged caution in promoting shellfish production. Yet shellfish play an important role in reducing the impact of nitrogen-rich runoff from industrial and agricultural processes. Although many strategies should be employed to prevent this contamination in the first place, is a "completely bare" ocean floor, devoid of life, really the preferable option relative to a rich, thriving ecosystem? An ecosystem that not only reduces the impacts of pollution but fosters an expansion of a vast array of life, to say nothing of being nutritious food for people?

To us, this feels eerily similar to the stance taken around ruminants. In fact, moose produce large amounts of methane and the Green Party in Sweden is now proposing that citizens should "shoot as many moose as possible and reduce the number of cattle," for the sake of the climate.[10] A myopic view of methane production is now casting doubt on the utility, if not sanity, of promoting more life on this planet. The misunderstanding and fear surrounding this topic are so potent that seemingly credible people are suggesting we should have less life on earth . . . so we can protect the other life on earth, and all to reduce the perceived danger of biologically sourced methane (which is a process that has occurred since the earliest days of life on earth). In one case, this is affecting the view of the natural state of grasslands and grazing animals; in the other, it deals with lynchpin organisms on the seafloor.

So where do all these exaggerated methane claims against cattle come from? Why does the Meatless Mondays campaign have memes saying that livestock production causes more GHG emissions than the entire transport sector? It all comes from a 2006 analysis by the Food and Agriculture Organization of the United Nations (FAO) called *Livestock's Long Shadow*. The report stated that livestock produce 18 percent of all GHG emissions, which was more than the transportation sector.

This number is circulated by the media constantly, even though the researchers have conceded it was an unfair assessment and have since reduced that figure. When UC Davis animal scientist Frank Mitloehner analyzed how the data was gathered, he found a striking methodological error. In the case of cattle, a full life cycle analysis was done on the industry. This means they looked at the feed production, transport of the feed, processing, transport to stores, and the like—everything from what the animal ate to how it ends up in a consumer's meal. There's a lot more going on here than cow burps.

More damningly, the same cradle-to-grave assessment was not conducted on the transportation sector. Only direct emissions from burning gasoline were calculated. Many other factors in the transportation industry contribute to GHG production, like how the cars or planes were made, how the metal was extracted, the energy required to run the factories, and how to transport and refine the oil. So while they did a full life cycle analysis on livestock, they did not do the same for transportation, unfairly leading the public to think that animal agriculture is worse than the transportation industry.

There is no full life cycle assessment on the total impact of the transportation industry worldwide. In the 2013 report the FAO calculated that worldwide all human activities (including fossil fuels) add up to about 6.9 gigatons a year, about 14.5 percent of all emissions, and that direct emissions from livestock were 2.3 gigatons, about 5 percent of global GHG emissions.

DIRECT VS LIFE CYCLE EMISSIONS

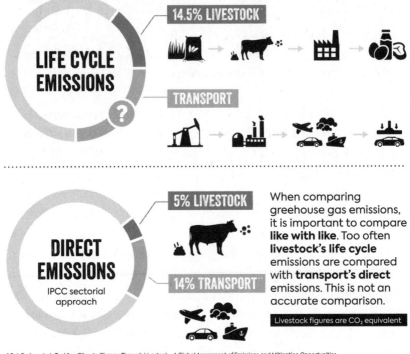

LIFE CYCLE EMISSIONS

14.5% LIVESTOCK*

TRANSPORT

DIRECT EMISSIONS
IPCC sectorial approach

5% LIVESTOCK

14% TRANSPORT**

When comparing greenhouse gas emissions, it is important to compare **like with like**. Too often **livestock's life cycle** emissions are compared with **transport's direct** emissions. This is not an accurate comparison.

Livestock figures are CO₂ equivalent

* P. J. Gerber et al., *Tackling Climate Change Through Livestock—A Global Assessment of Emissions and Mitigation Opportunities* (Rome: Food and Agriculture Organization of the United Nations, 2003), www.fao.org/3/a-i3437e.pdf.
** Rajendra K. Pachauri et al., *Climate Change 2014: Synthesis Report* (Geneva: Intergovernmental Panel on Climate Change, 2015), www.ipcc.ch/site/assets/uploads/2018/05/SYR_AR5_FINAL_full_wcover.pdf.

In the United States, the number might be lower than that worldwide figure. According to the EPA, all livestock only represents 3.9 percent of GHG emissions. Within the livestock category, beef cattle only represent 2 percent of total GHG emissions. (Another recent study put GHG emissions from cattle, including the production of feed, at 3.3 percent of greenhouse gas emissions in the US,[11] a number slightly higher than the EPA's.) Clearly, there are a lot of moving pieces here that make computing the actual percentages a challenge, but in any case, the number is *far* lower than the 18–51 percent[12] that many plant-based advocates report. The largest source of GHG emissions in the US comes from energy and transportation. These numbers are looking at emissions only for all industries and do not take into account any of the potential sequestration or net ecological benefit that cattle bring to the land.

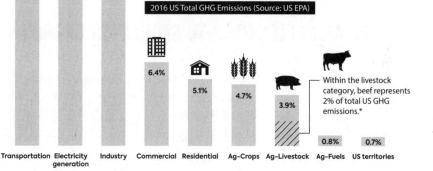

METHANE CLAIMS AGAINST CATTLE ARE OVERBLOWN

According the EPA, all livestock only represents 3.9% of the US GHG emissions, which is far lower than the 18–51% range many plant-based advocates report. The largest source of GHG emissions in the US comes from energy and transportation.

2016 US Total GHG Emissions (Source: US EPA)

Transportation 28.5%
Electricity generation 28.4%
Industry 21.6%
Commercial 6.4%
Residential 5.1%
Ag-Crops 4.7%
Ag-Livestock 3.9%
Ag-Fuels 0.8%
US territories 0.7%

Within the livestock category, beef represents 2% of total US GHG emissions.*

* "Agriculture Sector Emissions," Greenhouse Gas Emissions, United States Environmental Protection Agency, accessed December 31, 2019, www.epa.gov/ghgemissions/sources-greenhouse-gas-emissions#agriculture.

Why are the US livestock GHG emission numbers a smaller percentage contributor than the global numbers? A few reasons. We have more advanced agricultural practice here than in many other countries. Our cattle are also much more efficient at producing meat and milk than other countries. In the US one dairy cow can produce about twenty thousand pounds of milk a year. In Mexico you would need five cows to produce that much, and in India you'd need twenty.[13] Also, in less-developed countries, for example, there are more animals compared to cars and energy production, so the percentage of emissions from animals will be higher simply because there is less transportation and industry.

To further complicate this whole story, during the writing of this book, a new study was published showing that fertilizer plants emit a hundred times more methane than the industry previously reported.[14] Once this is folded into the GHG emissions data, it will be even clearer that synthetic chemical-driven industrial monocrop agriculture—which has brought us high yields at the expense of soil loss, ecosystem destruction, and intense GHG emissions—will no longer be acceptable as we move into the future.

This is all technical, sometimes counterintuitive material that is hotly debated. One point that is perhaps more universal is that it may be important to develop and expand smart methods to extract carbon from the atmosphere and store it somewhere.

HOW CAN CATTLE HELP TO SEQUESTER CARBON?

We can build expensive contraptions to capture carbon, but the energy required to produce and operate these seems exorbitantly high. This is not dissimilar to the misguided promise of "sustainable lab-grown meat." With innovation, we may in fact develop industrial methods of extracting and storing vast sums of atmospheric carbon in a manner that makes sense with regards to energy inputs (if you need to burn a "lot" of fossil fuels to try and sequester carbon, they may not pencil out as a net win). But what if there is a more elegant way of tackling this problem, one that favorably addresses many issues at once? To this end, we'd like to explain how cattle can be part of the solution.

When discussions of climate change crop up, it is often overlooked that healthy soils (which are part of a dynamic interaction between plants and animals) store carbon. Lots of it. Despite this, the current narrative on climate change implicates animals that emit GHG, and specifically cattle. It may be prudent to consider that holistically managed livestock are critical to systems that can build healthy soil *and* produce healthy food.

According to a paper in the *Journal of Soil and Water Conservation*, most agricultural soils have lost 30–70 percent of their soil organic carbon, which has led to a decrease in food production.[15] The majority of the damage when it comes to agricultural GHG emissions comes from plowing up fields for crop production—*not* belching cattle—and most of the opportunity for improvement in this area comes from no-till cropping practices. One paper that looked at the impacts agriculture has had on the Great Plains illustrates that the plowing of native grasslands peaking in the 1930s was the most devastating when it comes to carbon emissions. The researchers estimate that if only 25 percent of producers switch to no-till practices, there would be a 25 percent improvement in GHG emissions. If 100 percent switched, the improvement would increase to a whopping 80 percent.[16] And what if they also incorporated grazing animals into the mix? Then we'd be getting somewhere!

The earth holds approximately 3,170 gigatons (GT) of carbon (a gigaton is one billion metric tons). About 2,700 GT, or 80 percent of this, is found in soil. All the plants and animals on earth together constitute only 560 GT. Soil holds four times more carbon than trees and about three times more carbon than the atmosphere itself.[17]

Some estimates suggest that reversing climate change would require the removal of about 700 GT of carbon.[18] It would be impossible to plant enough trees to do this, and the oceans seem to suffer with more carbon, becoming more acidic. Our biggest opportunity is to sequester carbon in soil, which actually benefits biodiversity and can feed us with nutrient-dense food. Another important point is that the carbon in soil is actually the driving facilitator of helpful work—the cycling of nutrients.

Some exciting new research is being done looking at the impact and carbon cycle of well-managed cattle. In one recent study, researchers from Michigan State University tracked carbon in the soil in two different systems of raising beef cattle over four years, comparing the traditional feedlot system to a new method known as adaptive multi-paddock (AMP) grazing, where the cattle finished on grass were moved frequently to allow plants to recover and protect the soil. And although the feedlot system produced less total emissions (in terms of cow burps), the AMP system resulted in a net GHG *sink*. **The emissions in the finishing stage were more than completely offset by the amount of carbon sequestered in the**

ground. And it was not just a little bit of carbon but 3.59 metric tons of carbon per hectare, per year.[19]

Michigan State has also just completed (yet not published at the time of writing this book) a study showing the entire life cycle of 100 percent grass-fed beef at White Oak Pastures, a farm in Georgia, showing that the net total emissions were the equivalent of minus 3.5 kilograms of CO_2 per kilogram of fresh meat.[20] This is significant because not only is it better than conventional beef, pork, and chicken, it's also better than the claims of Beyond Burger and soybean production.

To see how this is possible, consider this graphic adapted from White Oak Pastures, a farm that uses regenerative agricultural practices:

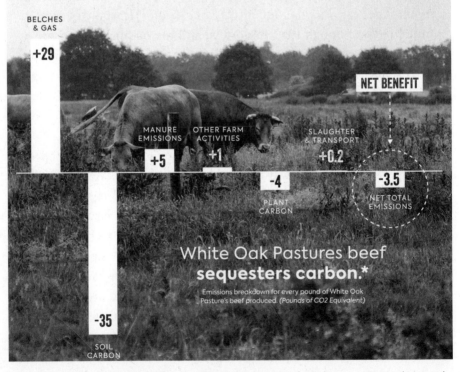

CATTLE CAN BENEFIT OUR CLIMATE

BELCHES & GAS
+29

NET BENEFIT

MANURE EMISSIONS
+5

OTHER FARM ACTIVITIES
+1

SLAUGHTER & TRANSPORT
+0.2

-4
PLANT CARBON

-3.5
NET TOTAL EMISSIONS

White Oak Pastures beef **sequesters carbon.***

Emissions breakdown for every pound of White Oak Pasture's beef produced. *(Pounds of CO2 Equivalent)*

-35
SOIL CARBON

J. E. Rowntree et al., "Ecosystem Impacts and Productive Capacity of a Multispecies Pastured Livestock System," *Frontiers in Sustainable Food Systems* (in review, 2020).

GRASS-FED BEEF VS OTHER PROTEIN

An independent **Life Cycle Analysis** found that for every Beyond Burger or Impossible Burger you eat, you'd have to eat one **White Oak Pastures** grass-fed beef burger to **offset your emissions.***

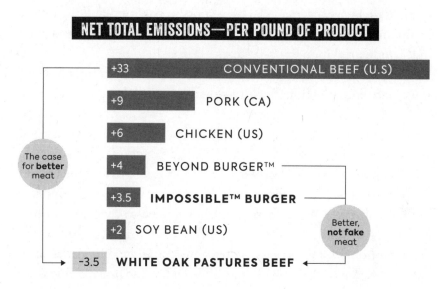

NET TOTAL EMISSIONS—PER POUND OF PRODUCT

+33	CONVENTIONAL BEEF (U.S)
+9	PORK (CA)
+6	CHICKEN (US)
+4	BEYOND BURGER™
+3.5	IMPOSSIBLE™ BURGER
+2	SOY BEAN (US)
-3.5	WHITE OAK PASTURES BEEF

The case for **better** meat

Better, **not fake** meat

* J. E. Rowntree et al., "Ecosystem Impacts and Productive Capacity of a Multispecies Pastured Livestock System," *Frontiers in Sustainable Food Systems* (in review, 2020).

Through the right practices, this farm's example illustrates that net carbon reduction and even sequestration is possible—and the key is healthy soil.

Another meta-analysis looking at carbon sequestration in soils from livestock grazing in several South American countries showed that grazing lands not only sequester carbon but also that the amount sequestered could partially or totally offset urban emissions. The researchers concluded that "the potential of grazing lands to sequester and store carbon should be reconsidered in order to improve assessments in future GHG inventory reports."[21] In other words, it's wrong to take a reductionistic view and blame grazing cattle for methane emissions. Instead, we need to consider the full picture and realize their impact is helping to sequester carbon.

As we write this book, there are several more papers coming out about how cattle can be a net carbon sink. The Savory Institute and other organizations are also starting to document other ecological outcomes from grazing animals, like water filtration rates, increase in plant diversity, decreases in bare spots in pastures, and the return of pollinators, birds, and other wildlife. None of this is happening in the industrial monocrop system.

Maybe you're still not convinced. You may be thinking, "But if we're trying to eliminate all this methane, shouldn't we eliminate all animals from our food system?" A study we mentioned in chapter six looked at the nutritional and environmental consequences of eliminating all livestock from the US food system. In this scenario, GHG emissions would decrease by only 2.6 percent, and the impact on our nutrient availability would be devastating. Because animals are more nutrient dense than plants, we'd need to eat a lot more to get the same nutrition. Overall calories would increase, our grain consumption would increase by ten times, and we'd be deficient in calcium, vitamins A and B12, and EPA, DHA, and arachidonic acid.

In short, we'd have more nutrition-related diseases. The researchers concluded, "When animals are allowed to convert some energy-dense, micronutrient-poor crops (e.g., grains) into more micronutrient-dense foods (meat, milk, and eggs), the food production system has enhanced capacity to meet the micronutrient requirements of the population."[22] What we take away from this is that even typical beef is a net win for our food system nutritionally, and if we improve our production and finish cattle in a well-managed system on grass, which helps dramatically reduce emissions, then it can benefit the environment as well.

If we're sincerely interested in cutting down on our GHG emissions, the solution is not to eliminate all animals from our food system. Livestock just needs to be managed in a better way.[23] It's not the *cow*, it's the *how*.

ELIMINATING MEAT WOULD DO MORE HARM THAN GOOD

A study found that if the entire US **eliminated all animal products**, GHG emissions would **only be reduced by 2.6%**, but would result in more overall calories consumed, increased carbohydrates, and would lead to **more nutrient deficiencies**, including calcium, vitamin B12, vitamin A, EPA, DHA and arachidonic acid.*

2.6%
US EMISSIONS DECREASE

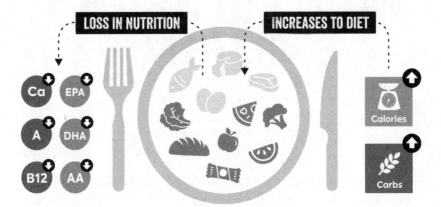

LOSS IN NUTRITION

INCREASES TO DIET

Ca EPA

A DHA

B12 AA

Calories

Carbs

* Robin R. White and Mary Beth Hall, "Nutritional and Greenhouse Gas Impacts of Removing Animals from US Agriculture," *PNAS* 114, no. 48 (November 28, 2017), www.pnas.org/content/114/48/E10301.

CHAPTER 10

AREN'T CATTLE INEFFICIENT WITH FEED?

Those who argue that eliminating animals from our food system is the only way to a sustainable future have good intentions but may be committing a serious oversight, not dissimilar to the McGovern commission's in our dietary recommendations. Let's walk through some of the concerns surrounding cattle:

- They're inefficient with feed.
- They take up too much land.
- They use too much water.

In the next three chapters we'll address each of these points directly and show you how there's more to the story than you might think. Then, we'll consider how well-managed cattle actually may benefit the land much more than monocrops.

DOESN'T IT TAKE TONS OF FEED TO PRODUCE A POUND OF BEEF?

After the climate change argument, the case against meat typically shifts to resource allocation. What food inputs are necessary to raise meat?

You may have heard an argument like this: "Our food supply is limited. Feeding available food to animals is inefficient and unethical. We should allocate it instead for people. Meat is an unsustainable luxury."

There's an often-regurgitated statistic that it takes twelve to twenty pounds of feed to produce a pound of beef.

If you recall, earlier in this section we mentioned that a key element to analyzing the relative sustainability of a given process is the net energy obtained compared to the net energy input. Here, however, there are many different calculations for feed-to-meat conversion (energy in versus energy out). But it all depends on how you define the word *feed*.[1]

Industrially produced monogastric farm animals like chicken and pork are fed a diet of primarily grain, which is grown on arable land that could be used to produce food for humans. (This is another mistake in DiCaprio's *Before the Flood*—chicken is actually *not* a better option than beef when considering inputs and outputs.) As ruminant animals, cattle can't handle a diet of 100 percent grain (sometimes referred to as "concentrates"). In fact, an overexposure to grain in too short a time can be fatal for a cow. Ruminants need a lower concentration of grain to keep them healthy, so most cattle, sheep, and goats' diets come from pasture, hay, cornstalks, and other "crop residues." These nonstarchy, fibrous plant materials can be "handled" one of three ways: as food for animals, as a composting matrix (which releases water vapor, methane, and CO_2, all greenhouse gases), or this material can go through the slow process of oxidation, which is the telltale sign of a damaged ecosystem.

LIVESTOCK TURN FOOD WE CAN'T EAT INTO PROTEIN

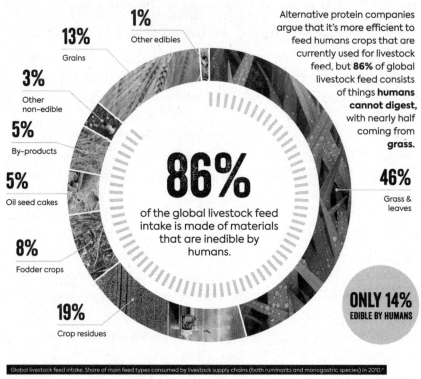

1%
Other edibles

13%
Grains

3%
Other non-edible

5%
By-products

5%
Oil seed cakes

8%
Fodder crops

19%
Crop residues

Alternative protein companies argue that it's more efficient to feed humans crops that are currently used for livestock feed, but **86%** of global livestock feed consists of things **humans cannot digest**, with nearly half coming from **grass**.

86%
of the global livestock feed intake is made of materials that are inedible by humans.

46%
Grass & leaves

ONLY 14%
EDIBLE BY HUMANS

Global livestock feed intake. Share of main feed types consumed by livestock supply chains (both ruminants and monogastric species) in 2010.*

* Anne Mottet, "Livestock: On Our Plates or Eating at Our Table? A New Analysis of the Feed/Food Debate," *Global Food Security* 14 (September 2017): 1–8, doi.org/10.1016/j.gfs.2017.01.001.

Now, in the case of chicken and pork, we are talking about a highly energy-intensive process that diverts what is ostensibly human food into animal food, but this is almost purely grains and legume products such as soybeans. With cattle, it's quite different. When looking at what only ruminants eat, the numbers are even lower for grain, at only 10–13 percent of the diet for cattle, globally. Grass and leaves makes up 57.4 percent of global ruminant feed rations. The rest is inedible by humans, like "crop residue" such as cornstalks.

While we're not necessarily advocating for feedlot beef, we also feel that typical beef has gotten a bad rap and that most people don't understand that the system really isn't as evil as you might think. Let's take a step back and look at the life of beef cattle. Contrary to what many people imagine, cattle do not spend their entire lives on a feedlot eating grain. Even typical (feedlot) cattle live the first half to two-thirds of their lives on pasture, eating grass and other forage. Some cattle can graze leftover cropland like cornfields that have been harvested, converting cornstalks and other crop "residues" into beef, with the added benefit of fertilizing that field with their manure as they clean up the field. Overgrazing is definitely an issue in many ranching operations, but we feel this is an opportunity to fix the system. In response to the "plants = good" and "meat = bad" paradigm, we'd like you to consider this question: Is overgrazing worse than industrial synthetic-chemical monocropping?

Regional variations also have a dramatic hand to play in this story. In situations where winters are harsh or land is sparse, supplementing cattle can improve their health. When cattle are given supplemental feed that is produced close to the farm for short periods when the animal doesn't have access to good grass, it can be part of a sustainable system. This is a process that has been used around the world for many years—for example, systems like Scotland's that go back hundreds, if not thousands, of years. Forage plants (cool-season grasses like fescue, for example) can also be stockpiled and can greatly reduce the cost of supplemental feed. In some areas these forages are allowed to grow in late summer and into fall without grazing, and then grazed in late fall or early winter. Cattle will graze through a bit of snow, and some of these cool-season grasses like fescue stay green longer and maintain nutrient levels for cattle well into cold months. In this system, producers can avoid the fossil fuels and labor costs of putting up feed or buying feed.

Unless they are "grass finished," beef cattle will spend the last four to six months at a feedlot where they're harvested at around eighteen months of age. To fully understand the inputs and outputs of this system, let's look at what cattle eat when on a feedlot. When cattle reach the feedlot, much of their diet comes from by-products from the food industry like grain leftovers from distilleries and other field residue (e.g., cornstalks, corn gluten, soybean hulls, cottonseed meal, almond husks, and beet pulp). These inedible by-products provide nourishment for the cattle that would otherwise go to waste.

The amount of feed needed for an animal is called the feed conversion ratio. A recent life cycle analysis calculated that the amount of grain required to produce one pound of boneless beef is 2.6 pounds. The ratio of pork is about 3.5:1, chicken 2:1, and many farmed fish like salmon are 1.3:1.[2]

Over their life span, typical cattle only get 10 percent of their diet from grain.[3] This means that about 90 percent of the feed for beef is inedible by humans. Let's ruminate on that for a moment: Cattle convert grass and other nutrient-poor food into nutrient-dense food for humans. This is something ruminants are really good at doing. They're upcycling nutrients! One study found that "cattle need only 0.6 kg of protein from edible feed to produce 1 kg of protein in milk and meat. Cattle thus contribute directly to global food security."[4]

CATTLE ARE MORE THAN FOOD

Although it is reasonable to ask hard questions regarding food production when we face a global population surging toward ten billion people, we must also remember ruminants provide much more than food. Only 42 percent of an animal's live weight is retail muscle and ground meats, but that hardly means the rest of the animal goes to "waste." A whopping 44 percent of the animal is turned into other products that we in America aren't eating. The hide becomes leather, and the bones, fat, and intestines are processed into other items like soap, fertilizer, pharmaceuticals, and pet food. Eliminating animals from our food system would mean more synthetic substitutes made from fossil fuels. In America, we tend not to eat organ meats (offal), but many other countries have a high demand for liver, heart, tongue, tail, and kidneys, which account for 12 percent of the live weight from cattle. In Asia, economics and culinary tradition have maintained a particularly high demand for offal, and many consider muscle meat to be too bland. Traditional Mexican dishes like *putzaze* (tripe and liver with tomatoes,) *lengua* (tongue), and *menudo norteño* (tripe soup) are still highly valued.[5]

THE MANY PRODUCTS FROM CATTLE

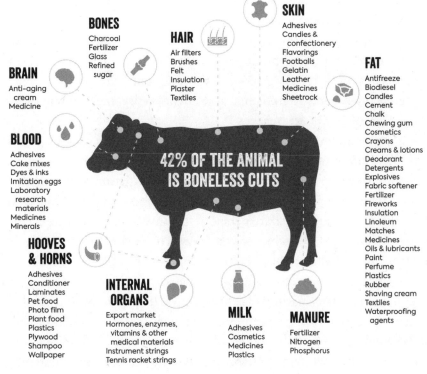

BONES
Charcoal
Fertilizer
Glass
Refined sugar

HAIR
Air filters
Brushes
Felt
Insulation
Plaster
Textiles

SKIN
Adhesives
Candies & confectionery
Flavorings
Footballs
Gelatin
Leather
Medicines
Sheetrock

BRAIN
Anti-aging cream
Medicine

FAT
Antifreeze
Biodiesel
Candles
Cement
Chalk
Chewing gum
Cosmetics
Crayons
Creams & lotions
Deodorant
Detergents
Explosives
Fabric softener
Fertilizer
Fireworks
Insulation
Linoleum
Matches
Medicines
Oils & lubricants
Paint
Perfume
Plastics
Rubber
Shaving cream
Textiles
Waterproofing agents

BLOOD
Adhesives
Cake mixes
Dyes & inks
Imitation eggs
Laboratory research materials
Medicines
Minerals

42% OF THE ANIMAL IS BONELESS CUTS

HOOVES & HORNS
Adhesives
Conditioner
Laminates
Pet food
Photo film
Plant food
Plastics
Plywood
Shampoo
Wallpaper

INTERNAL ORGANS
Export market
Hormones, enzymes, vitamins & other medical materials
Instrument strings
Tennis racket strings

MILK
Adhesives
Cosmetics
Medicines
Plastics

MANURE
Fertilizer
Nitrogen
Phosphorus

Adapted from "Where's the (Not) Meat? Byproducts from Beef and Pork Production," United States Department of Agriculture.

Since these "by-products" are used by other industries, it's not accurate to calculate the bones, hide, and exported offal into the feed conversion ratio and claim cattle are inefficient at converting feed to meat.

Now, many feedlot beef systems have waste management and other issues, but it's important to point out that a lot of the criticisms of this system are also inaccurate. When we consider the energy inputs and outputs of a complex food system, well-managed grass-fed beef is ideal. Far from being an ecological catastrophe, it may literally be close to a "free lunch." But compared to many other foods, even beef finished on corn is a much better choice. Beyond Burger is one famous plant-based meat substitute that's gotten large amounts of funding. But is this a healthier product than grass-finished beef, and is it really better for the environment? The main ingredients are pea protein isolate and canola oil. Do you think that chemically sprayed monocropped peas and canola fields are causing less harm than a field of grass-fed cattle on land we can't crop, increasing biodiversity and soil health? Is this product increasing or decreasing biodiversity and soil health? They aren't even using organic ingredients, and nutritionally, this is a pale comparison to a real beef burger.

If it is unethical to allocate agricultural products such as grains to the feeding of animals, why is there no concerted effort to block the use of these commodities for alcohol production? Said another way, why no picket lines around distilleries, breweries, and wineries?

From an animal welfare perspective, think about the living conditions of typical CAFO chickens and pigs. They're indoors 100 percent of the time, under artificial lights, living in tight quarters. Cattle, on the other hand, are free ranging for most of their lives, in sunlight, eating a diet that's natural for their bodies. If they do go to a feedlot, they're still outdoors and can move relatively freely. This makes large ruminants, like cattle, a better choice than other land animals for the majority of human protein. And as we discussed in the nutrition chapter, the meat from ruminant animals is also far more nutritious than chicken or pork. From this perspective, it is baffling that Hollywood celebrities, politicians, and political action committees could think that pork or chicken production is a "win" compared to the ruminant/grasslands system. As a reminder, cattle are upcycling nutrients we can't eat into nutrients we can—and as we'll explore next, they're largely doing it on land that isn't suitable for crops anyway.

Pork and poultry production have existed in quite different ways up until recent times. Throughout history, humans fed chickens and pigs our "waste." It wasn't until the past fifty years that grains began to be grown specifically for animal feed.

Anyone who has had backyard chickens knows that they devour greens and other kitchen scraps. Eating chicken was considered a luxury until relatively recently. Worldwide, poultry consumption has risen over 418 percent, while beef consumption across the world is only up 3 percent. Why is this? Chicken is cheap to produce under our current systems, which rely on cheap oil. What might happen to the price of chicken—and, indeed, of fake meat products like lab meat—if the price of energy goes up? Grazing animals, meanwhile, rely on photosynthesis.

Humans have historically kept pigs in either a free-roaming situation or closer to us as our living condensed into settlements, and they did not compete with humans for food. (Off the coast of New England, there were numerous "hog islands" where pigs would freely live, and folks would just go hunt a pig when they needed it.)[6] As free-roaming domesticated animals, pigs thrived in woodland areas, eating fallen nuts and "rooting" for mushrooms, tubers, and small animals like mice and rabbits. As prolific reproducers and fast weight gainers that provide tasty meat and fat, pigs have been an important source of nourishment for many cultures. Ironically, one of the only foods common to all "Blue Zones," areas noted for significant health and longevity, is pork. In more densely populated areas, pigs lived closer to humans as "garbage disposals" that literally ate our waste. Yes, sorry to gross you out, pigs can eat human poop. In fact, in China and Korea a family of four humans could feed four young pigs on around four and a half pounds of human waste and eight ounces of garbage each day.[7] Pigs played an important role in medieval Paris for, of all things, sanitation. In fifteenth-century Ireland it was common to keep a pig primarily on food scraps, then process the animal as the weather got colder to provide nutrient-dense meat and vital fat in the winter. Pigs were their savings accounts. If cattle are upcyclers, pigs are recyclers.

Feeding pigs food scraps seems like a win-win, yet it's made virtually impossible in many places because of government regulations. While the USDA estimates that between 30 and 40 percent of food is wasted in the US, we foolishly grow large amounts of grain on land that we could be using for human food to feed to pigs. Rules vary state by state, and some farmers are converting food waste to pig food, but in general, because of the equipment and licensing requirements, many producers find that it's simply easier to buy grain from outside companies. Because oil is currently cheap, grain is subsidized, margins are slim, and regulations make it difficult (or in some areas impossible) to feed pigs food waste. The main way pigs are fed, as of today, is primarily with grain.[8]

According to the Food and Agriculture Organization, one-third of all food produced, about 1.3 billion tons, is lost or wasted.[9] The largest percentage of waste comes from roots and tubers and fruit and vegetables. Some of this waste is not fit for animal consumption, but since pigs have survived for thousands of years on recycled human food waste, clearly we can do better than the current system. Leftover bread, dairy, and produce from retail and catering could easily be fed to pigs, freeing up valuable arable land for crops for humans. Several countries in Asia, including Japan and South Korea, are already encouraging producers to feed pigs food waste, and selling it in stores as "eco-pork" for a premium. Feeding pigs food waste is cheaper for farmers because they don't have to purchase grain (feed is 60–75 percent of the cost of raising pigs), has a lower carbon footprint because grain doesn't have to travel from faraway places to the farms, and frees up precious agricultural land for human feed.

Part of the controversy surrounding the feeding of animal by-products to farm animals comes from the spread of BSE (bovine spongiform encephalopathy, or mad cow disease). Cattle and other ruminants are not omnivores like chickens and pigs, and they cannot thrive on the variety of food waste that pigs can. There is no evidence that feeding pigs, and even chickens, our leftover properly treated food waste, is unsafe.[10]

CHAPTER 11

DON'T CATTLE TAKE UP TOO MUCH LAND?

You may have heard that livestock take up two-thirds of our agricultural land. The Meatless Mondays campaign pronounces an even more sensational figure: "75% of Earth's Agricultural Land." It makes a great meme, implying that if we only removed these inefficient, "land hogging" animals, we'd free up more space for soybeans, zucchini, and lettuce. You may have also heard the often-quoted stats that one acre of land can produce 50,000 pounds of tomatoes, 53,000 pounds of potatoes, and 30,000 pounds of carrots, but only 250 pounds of beef. That sounds pretty wasteful, right? Why would we bother raising beef when we can be so productive with crops?

There are two problems with this argument. The first is that we're not comparing apples to apples—that is, we're not comparing foods of the same nutrient value. As you read in the nutrition section, animal protein calories are much more valuable than carbohydrate calories to humans. You would need to eat about six hundred calories worth of beans and rice (two cups of black beans and a half cup of brown rice) to get the same amount of protein you can get from only 160 calories of beef (3.5oz of sirloin), not to mention B12 and heme iron. So as we consider what can be raised on equal amounts of land, let's be sure to compare foods of equal nutrients, not just overall calories. We've said it before and we'll say it again: we don't need more calories in our food system; we need more nutrients.

Second, and what is the most important takeaway from this chapter, is that most of the world's agricultural land *cannot* grow tomatoes, potatoes, and carrots (or other crops). Think about all the brittle, dry, rocky, hilly landscapes across the planet. In order to grow large fields of crops, you need fertile soil, enough rainfall or access to water for irrigation, relatively flat land, and the infrastructure to till, harvest, and process the crops that aren't eaten right away. Well-managed cattle and other ruminants can thrive on land where we can't grow crops, and they are beneficial to the land. There's much more land suitable to grazing than there is land suitable for cropping. In effect, cattle (and ruminants at large) are not competing for space that could otherwise yield crops. If properly managed, they are playing a vital ecological role *and* converting food that cannot be used by humans (forage) to food that is indeed usable.

The Food and Agriculture Organization of the United Nations estimates that approximately one-third of the earth's agricultural land is considered suitable for growing crops (arable land and permanent crops). Of this potentially arable land, currently one-third (1.5 billion hectares) is in use.[1] This sounds like there's lots of room for more crops, right? Well, of the remaining potential cropland, nearly half is currently in forest (areas that were in fact once cropland, but returned to a largely wild state, ironically because of a decrease in total land needs as a consequence of the Green Revolution and intensive farming practices), 12 percent is protected, and 3 percent is already taken up by cities.[2]

While so many people are blaming conversion of the rainforest for grazing and soy production (some of this is legitimate, which we will address later), a bigger problem in the US is the conversion of grassland into cropland, which destroys habitat and releases carbon. In Iowa farmers are being paid a few dollars per acre to either practice no-till farming or convert their cropland to pasture. If the US Congress passes strict limits on GHG emissions, farmers stand to earn much more than this to store carbon.[3] Private companies are also jumping on board, seeking business that heavily emits carbon to invest in a program that pays farmers well to practice carbon-friendly farming.[4]

Approximately 60 percent of the world's agricultural land is grazing land.[5] Much of this land is not suitable for growing crops and is in fact appropriate only for some type of grazing, whether that be by cows, camels, bison, or goats. In many parts of the world

NOT ALL LAND CAN BE CROPPED

Removing cattle **doesn't mean that we'll free up more land** for crop production. More than 60% of agricultural land globally is pasture and rangeland that is **too rocky, steep, and/or arid** to support cultivated agriculture—**yet this land can support cattle and protein upcycling.***

60%

Ice sheet & polar desert	Temperate broadleaf forest	Mediterranean vegetation	Xeric shrubland	Grass savanna	Tropical rainforest
Tundra	Temperate steppe	Monsoon forest	Dry steppe	Tree savanna	Alpine tundra
Taiga	Subtropical rainforest	Arid desert	Semiarid desert	Subtropical dry forest	Montane forest

* "Livestock on Grazing Lands" in *Livestock & the Environment: Meeting the Challenge* (FAO), accessed December 31, 2019, www.fao.org/3/x5304e/x5304e03.htm.

raising grazing livestock is one of the only ways people can survive. And while overgrazing is an issue, we will explore later why the pivotal issue is not the number of animals on the land but how they are managed. Again, it's not the *cow*, it's the *how*.

But we still have good cropland left, right? Well, not all cropland is of the same quality, and cropland can't grow *every* crop. For example, large areas in North Africa can only grow olive trees. This land is counted as "suitable for crops," even though only one type of crop can thrive there. According to the Food and Agriculture Organization, about 36 percent of our planet's land surface is considered arable,[6] but only 3 percent of it is considered prime cropland.[7] There are multiple factors that come into play when considering the usability of cropland, such as whether the location is suitable for crops dependent on rainfall or requires irrigation. Water is a huge limiting factor. If an area has limited water, then it probably doesn't make sense to be growing crops that need heavy irrigation, even if the land is nice and flat and empty.

In the Democratic Republic of Congo, nearly 50 percent of the land is only suitable for growing cassava, and less than 3 percent can support wheat production.[8] But is there enough demand for cassava? Do they have the infrastructure to export surplus cassava? Can they store the excess? Is nutrient-poor cassava (high in starch, low in protein and micronutrients) a crop that most humans should really be eating a ton of? There are also issues with the infrastructure to properly process and store cassava. Will there be a huge demand in the future for cassava? If the land can only grow a product that not many people want (or should be eating), then is it truly valuable when it's used exclusively as cropland?

Many developing countries like India simply don't have the infrastructure to transport and store surplus crops, and are highly susceptible to weather-related disasters, which then put their crops at risk of rotting. With weather patterns becoming more unpredictable, farming is much trickier. In the northeast US summers used to receive a steady rainfall that was perfect for vegetable production. However, now we're seeing more drought,[9] followed by more intense rainfalls. Even though precipitation totals may be similar to years past, the quality of the rain has shifted in an unfavorable way, forcing farmers to change how they farm. Because we no longer have a relatively predictable, steady rainfall in the growing season, most vegetable farmers in this area now need to rely much more heavily on irrigation than they once did.

Of the 1.8 billion hectares of cropland left to exploit, most of this land is concentrated in just seven countries: Brazil, the Democratic Republic of the Congo, Sudan, Angola, Argentina, Colombia, and Bolivia.[10] South Asia and North Africa have virtually no cropland left at all. As soil-depleting monocropping expands in developing countries, economic pressure on these areas won't favor regenerative farming techniques that build the soil. This means that the more we "megacrop," the more soil degradation happens. As soil health fails, so will the amount of land that we have to farm. Yields can temporarily be maintained with chemical fertilizers, but this is a dead end for soil health.

As we intimated earlier, it's helpful to think of soil as a bank account. Annual crops (corn, soy, wheat, and most vegetables) cost a lot of "money," in the form of nutrients. You can't just continue to harvest or "withdraw" from your bank account. Soil in an industrial cropping system needs deposits, either from mined minerals and chemicals or from natural inputs. The problem with relying on minerals (a finite resource) is that the more you use, the more you need. The earth is not limitless in its stores of resources. We simply don't have endless supplies of cropland, oil, or phosphorus to maintain artificially increased yields. This means the cost of farming will inevitably increase as resources become scarcer. In addition, it's simply not enough to just input the basics of nitrogen, phosphorus, and potassium without paying attention to the other nutrients and life that healthy soil needs.

Many traditional cultures—if they were to adopt the nutrition and food production guidelines popularized within affluent developed nations—would be incapable of producing *any* of their own nutrition. They would be entirely dependent on row crops raised thousands of miles away. And as we've seen, row crops likely have an expiration date.

Ruminants like cattle, bison, goats, and sheep convert grass we can't eat to protein, fatty acids, vitamins, and minerals that we can. And they are doing this on land we can't use for cropping, contributing to food security.[11]

HOW ARE WE USING OUR CROPLAND?

Human sprawl consumes remarkable swaths of valuable space that ought to be used for growing crops. Think about all the expanding suburban areas, the cookie-cutter houses, strip malls, and chain coffee shops—suburbia is built on what was once prime farmland.

One could make a compelling ecological case for megacities as they clearly furnish us with efficiency in terms of centralization of populations and resources.[12] Yet urban planners are reticent to alter their iconic skylines, often bending to the political will of folks claiming to be advancing the cause of "affordable housing"—so long as it's not too close to their zip code. With the proliferation of the internet and telecommuting, there's less of a desire to live in crowded cities, and folks don't really need to physically be in the office anymore.

The first wave of this sprawl in the US coincided with the advent of a miraculous invention that capitalized on the availability of cheap oil, expanded highway systems, and ubiquitous access to transportation and freedom: the car. People no longer had to live where they worked; they could live in a nearby city or suburb. There are pluses and minuses to any development, but the modern iteration of this commute means folks in the Bay Area spend more than three hours per day in their cars.

Today, thanks to the Internet, lots of folks want their piece of a few acres out in the hinterlands. Country living comes at a price, however. The value of "farmland" has skyrocketed—not for its utility as a resource that could feed us, but as a place for new housing.

McMansion expansions occupy land once worked by small- to medium-sized farmers, leaving either no farming or a consolidation toward huge monopolies. Whether we are talking about a real estate boom spurred by dodgy government-backed lending policies (as was the case in the 2008 mortgage crisis) or the urban flight from states such as California, New York, and New Jersey, the net effect is a loss of some of the most accessible farmland in the world.[13] Cabbage and broccoli are great, but compared to selling land to developers, they don't really pay the bills. Now, this might be a good thing for well-off individuals and to alleviate congested traffic grids. But once farmland has been paved over it is unlikely to see the light of day until well after the collapse of humanity.

The topics of sustainability, climate change, and feeding the world are critically important. But where our cropland is "going" and what cropland is actually used for are frequently ignored, with more politically charged topics such as animal husbandry taking center stage.

The farming of biofuels also directly competes with humans for food acres. While it doesn't often make the front page, 37.5 percent of corn acreage in the US is used for producing fuel ethanol.[14] This should be an issue that unifies the whole political spectrum. Although the research is not conclusive, the net energy gain from ethanol production ranges from negative to slightly positive. This might be why the farmers who grow corn for ethanol drive tractors that run on diesel or gasoline, not ethanol. This is a greenwashed boondoggle that costs more energy than it provides (one of our criteria for assessing the validity of a given practice) and is entirely supported by government subsidies. The government takes tax money, pays it to farmers to produce not food but ethanol, and the whole process consumes more energy than it produces. Paying people to dig and fill holes could arguably be more beneficial—at least they'd get some exercise and sunshine.

If dwindling space weren't enough of a problem, as we've learned, modern industrial farming practices are ruining the cropland we have. About one-third of the global agricultural land has been degraded,[15] and more than half this land is so damaged that farmers have no obvious means to restore it. Erosion, soil compaction, and nutrient loss from intensive mechanized chemical farming all contribute to the degradation of soil.[16]

In dry areas the problem is even worse, with approximately 70 percent of the land degraded.[17] Overgrazing is part of the reason for this, but this is a management issue, not a problem inherent in raising animals. What we will propose is that the judicious application of grazing animals may in fact be a route to rehabilitating damaged farmland.

HOW CAN WE REHABILITATE OUR LAND?

There are ways of improving soil quality with "green manure"— essentially, growing plants to plow them back into the soil so they can enrich the earth and serve as mulch. A cover crop, like clover, feeds the soil biology while also preventing erosion by wind and rain while the land is not being utilized for a cash crop. The resulting microbial activity from these crops also increases the availability of other vital minerals that crops need to thrive and provides habitat for beneficial insects. Cover crops are also being used in between rows of crops to prevent bare soil. Farmers can also graze livestock over cover crops.

Often, when farmers choose to plant cover crops, a portion of their land is temporarily taken out of production. It also costs money to buy the seeds. It may not be economically feasible for farmers to use this method in all regions.

Another proposed solution by those who advocate for "veganic" agriculture is the use of algae fertilizers. But when you analyze how algae is produced, you'll find it actually requires more inputs and energy than many realize. Large amounts of nitrogen and phosphorus are needed to keep algae alive, and those inputs have to come from somewhere. These algae systems don't scale easily, and it's also important to consider that importing algae from off the farm is far from a closed-loop system. That poses an economical problem for most farmers, when compared to generating their own fertilizers by using animals on-site. And how will the algae get to the farm?

Farmers can spread compost on the soil to capture more carbon. In addition, no-till agriculture systems are another solution receiving a lot of attention. Instead of deeply plowing soil, farmers will slice a narrow slit with disc seeds or seedlings, thereby not stirring up the soil and releasing carbon. No-till can significantly reduce the amount of nitrogen farmers need to apply to their soil and reduce soil erosion, but it does often increase the amount of herbicides needed. Producers touting the term "no till" should be questioned about their chemical inputs and other off-farm inputs, as the impact on the soil biology can be devastating.

No matter the technique, the main idea we're trying to get across is this: by far the best thing a farmer can do is increase soil biology, which is what's necessary to make minerals bioavailable to plants. A better, faster, and more regenerative solution to those listed above is to incorporate animals. Animals can graze on some of these nutrient-dense "green manure" crops while producing healthy meat or milk. Think of ruminants as four-legged speed composters. Joel Salatin of Polyface Farm told Diana in an interview that animals are like a flywheel compared to a compost pile. They break down the organic matter faster, especially in arid environments, without large amounts of water and without collection or redistribution. Their manure, urine, and saliva all contain bacteria that become part of the soil biome, so they increase the amount of nutrients available to plants.

In nature animals' gut flora and the earth's soil microbes are a circle. They're not separate systems. Moreover, using ruminants to graze down cover crops and then later crop residues can eliminate the need to use herbicides. Their manure is fertilizer, which helps activate the soil biology and reduces the need for external sources of nitrogen, phosphorus, and potassium, the three main components in chemical fertilizers. No oil or expensive human labor is required to synthesize or disperse the fertilizer from ruminants in a well-managed system.

According to the Food and Agriculture Organization, about 60–70 percent of all agricultural land is best suited to grazing.[18] Determining how many cattle can be supported by land is difficult because each landscape is dramatically different. What works in Vermont is completely different from what works in Nevada or southern Mexico or northern China. In Massachusetts, where Diana lives, the general recommendation is five hundred to eight hundred pounds of animal per acre of average land. This means a 1,200-pound cow requires about two acres of pasture, and because the environment is so humid, the water footprint of cattle in this region is very low, averaging about thirty gallons per pound of boneless beef (this will become clearer in the next chapter). One thing New England is really good at is growing pasture!

In chapter sixteen we'll go through the numbers and illustrate that, contrary to what many will assume, we do have the acreage to grass-finish all the beef cattle in the US. As soil health improves, so does water retention and the amount and quality of the pasture. With good management techniques like intensive grazing, the "carrying capacity" of the land is increased, meaning more cattle can be placed on the same amount of land.

What do we mean by well-managed cattle? Let's remember the Grassworld example from chapter seven. In a pasture, there are a variety of different types of grasses, forbs, wildflowers, and other plants. If the animal has access to the same area of land, day in and day out, it will pick its favorite plant variety and eat it down to nothing, killing the roots. This type of management is often called "continuous grazing." In this system, the more desirable plants can become overgrazed, allowing fewer desirable species to grow in their place. Unwanted grasses take over, and the cow is less likely to eat them. Overgrazing also leads to bare soil, loss of biodiversity both underground and above ground, increased soil compaction and erosion, and less carbohydrate reserves.

From a cattle health perspective, this is also not a good system because if there are parasites in their manure, these can easily be digested by the rest of the herd, causing an infestation. In the wild, herd animals are constantly moving owing to predator pressure, and they're followed by flocks of birds that pick out any parasites. The presence of predators keeps their numbers in check to prevent the herd population from growing out of control, and also keeps the pastures from being overgrazed. Of course, we don't need to keep a pack of hungry wolves on the farm in order to mimic this; electric fencing does a fantastic job. (And should Leonardo DiCaprio ever run a sustainable farm, *this* is the place to introduce chickens!) The number of animals per acre and frequency of rotation depends on a number of factors, and depending on the location, there are many goals to improving the ecosystem with cattle, like increasing ground cover, increasing forage, and repairing the water cycle.

When we look at various types of intensive cattle management, where the animals are put on a small piece of pasture for a short amount of time, then moved frequently, we can produce a lot more beef than in more conventional "continuous grazing" systems. Joel Salatin of Polyface Farms in Virginia calls this "mob grazing" and has calculated two acres for keeping a cow and producing a calf to finish for beef. Another framework put forth by the Savory Institute is holistic management, which considers multiple factors including land, animals, precipitation, and the farm's financial goals—and cattle can be an important tool in this process. The point is, not all grass-fed animals are really being managed for the best soil and animal health. Keeping them moving often is key.

There has been an interesting narrative around this whole topic that paints a false dichotomy. We either have plants or animals, and never the twain shall meet. We will look at the reasons behind this false dichotomy in the ethics section, but it's worth mentioning that the main opponents of animal-inclusive agriculture appear to have ignored how farms functioned before the Green Revolution. The reality is ruminants and crops can be grown on the livestock and cropland can be reintegrated where livestock either rotate through fields to graze covers and residues or are part of mixed-use systems. Some examples are called "pasture cropping" and "no-kill cropping." A lot of beef producers in the corn belt of the US graze their cattle on corn stalk residues, and in the southern Great Plains winter wheat is integrated with stocker cattle. Such systems improve yields and nearly eliminate the need for herbicides and fertilizers. Simplistic "land footprint" statistics don't tell us anything about the suitability of the land, multifunctional use, and quality of use (i.e., is this system building soil or degrading it?).

Instead of dictating that everyone in the world must eat less meat to save the planet, what if we stopped or dramatically reduced our intake of animals that eat grain and instead started eating more animals that eat grass? And what if those grass-eating animals were managed in a way that improved soil health and increased the capacity of land to produce more and better food? As counterintuitive as it may seem, from a nutritional standpoint, we'd be better off, as red meat from ruminants is nutritionally superior to poultry, grains, and even legume products. From a land-use perspective, it makes more sense to use grazing land instead of leaving it fallow. Also, cattle aren't the only animals that thrive on pastureland. In certain areas, it may make more sense to raise goats, bison, or camels, depending on the type of climate and vegetation/terrain. Wildlife like bees also need healthy, diverse pastures to thrive. This is where both authors feel that meat-phobic direction of global "sustainability plus health" dietary guidelines is incredibly dangerous, especially because they're written by people who have the privilege to push away a nutrient-dense food like meat (when many do not) and seem to have very little understanding of the multitude of benefits grazing animals have in a truly sustainable food system.

What about the Amazon rainforest that's being burned down for cattle? We have an extensive blog post by Lauren Manning that addresses this specific topic. In short, we obviously don't condone the burning of rainforest specifically for grazing. But that's not really what's happening. The US currently does not accept beef imports from Brazil, so protesting the burning of the Amazon by not eating beef would do nothing. This is a policy issue, not a cattle issue. See www.sacredcow.info/blog/the-amazon-fires-are-a-policy-issue-not-a-livestock-issue-heres-why.

CHAPTER 12

DON'T CATTLE DRINK TOO MUCH WATER?

As part of the Meatless Mondays campaign, every NYC school will have propaganda displayed claiming how horrible animals are for our health and the environment. One common narrative that makes for great, simplistic posters for school children is that it takes ten full bathtubs of water to produce a quarter-pound burger.

But upon closer examination of the methodology of these water calculations, a more complicated picture emerges. It turns out that most of the water attributed to the water footprint of cattle is the rain that would have fallen on the pasture, whether or not the animals were there.

What cattle need for drinking water is a very small percentage of the water calculation. Let us explain . . .

With any study examining water usage, it's important to know what exactly we're measuring. Types of water measured include green water, blue water, and gray water.

Green water is precipitation that is stored in the soil or rests on top of the soil or plants. Eventually, this water evaporates or the

BEEF ISN'T A WATER HOG

Most of the droplets below represent "green water," or **natural rainfall**.* "Blue water" represents water that has been sourced from surface or groundwater resources. **Beef requires only 280 gallons**** of "blue water" per pound, which is **less than** the amount required to produce a pound of avocados, walnuts, or sugar. Gray water is the volume of water required to dilute pollutants.

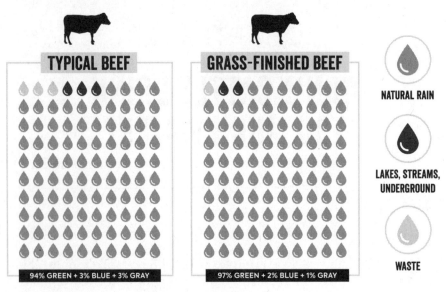

* Mesfin M. Mekonnen and Arjen Y. Hoekstra, "The Green, Blue, and Grey Water Footprint of Farm Animals and Animal Products," Value of Water Research Report Series 48, UNESCO-IHE (2010).
** C. Alan Rotz et al., "Environmental Footprints of Beef Cattle Production in the United States," *Agricultural Systems* 169 (February 2019): 1–13, doi.org/10.1016/j.agsy.2018.11.005.

crops take it up. Blue water is fresh surface and groundwater—what's found in lakes, rivers, and aquifers. Gray water is something else altogether. According to the Water Footprint Network,

> The grey water footprint of a product is an indicator of freshwater pollution that can be associated with the production of a product over its full supply chain. It is defined as the volume of freshwater that is required to assimilate the load of pollutants based on natural background concentrations and existing ambient water quality standards. It is calculated as the volume of water that is required to dilute pollutants to such an extent that the quality of the water remains above agreed water quality standards.[1]

So depending on what you're measuring, beef can either look fantastic or like a water hog. In typical cattle production, the green water number is about 92 percent of the total water calculation.[2] This means 92 percent of the water attributed to beef production is rain that would have fallen even if the cattle weren't alive. In grass-finished beef, the green water number is closer to 97–98 percent. There are some studies that actually show "typical beef" as using less water than grazing cattle—because when you use the green water methodology, feedlot-finished animals have higher hanging weights and a shorter life span than grass-finished animals, and therefore need less feed over their lifetimes to produce more beef. The problem, though, is that this feed for feedlots often requires irrigation—meaning blue water. And blue water is what's critical, not green water.[3] The water for a grass-fed animal is nearly all rain that would have fallen anyway, whether or not there were cattle on that field, and whether or not they ate the grass. As you can now see, it's critical to understand how the researchers derive their numbers!

A recent life cycle analysis study showed it takes only 280 gallons per pound of beef.[4] Some estimates put water usage for grass-finished beef closer to fifty to one hundred gallons per pound to produce.[5] The discrepancies in estimates are attributable to the very landscapes in which they are calculated. Factors such as humidity, temperature, and how long the animal lived dramatically affect the real story on water usage.[6]

Additionally, properly managed cattle (and other ruminants) increase benefits of green water by enhancing the ability of the soil to retain water. Interestingly, this is accomplished primarily because there's more soil carbon in well-managed pastures. The rainwater associates with the carbon and minerals in the soil, making more of it available longer and thus facilitating more grass growth.

A water footprint also doesn't tell us anything about whether the water source is in critical danger. Is the feed grown in a region of the Ogallala where the water level is dropping, or where it's being sustainably recharged? We don't know that info from a water footprint.[7] What percentage of the animal's feed is grain that was irrigated grain, and what percentage is crop residues that are essentially waste products, which would otherwise be discarded?

Also not calculated into the water argument are the benefits well-managed grazing animals have on the overall health of the land by improving soil biology. On hard, compacted land, rainfall runs off instead of being absorbed by the soil. If there's no cover and just exposed topsoil, rain can also wash lots of topsoil into nearby rivers. In a well-managed grazing system, the soil absorbs rainfall like a sponge and exposes the roots to water. This is especially critical in dry environments where there's little rain to begin with. This benefit can't be calculated using reductionist thinking. You must look at the entire system.

About 30 percent of what cattle consume is actually returned directly to the ecosystem through urine and manure, which adds beneficial nutrients and microbes to grasslands. If you recall from the Grassworld example, something needs to be eating the grasses in order for the grass to biologically break down instead of oxidize, particularly in a dry area, where many cattle graze. In a brittle landscape, rainfall is able to penetrate the top layer of soil only when there is sufficient microbial activity underground. Luckily, cattle and other ruminants can help keep grasslands healthy by biologically breaking down plants, enhancing water retention and carbon sequestration. Their manure is only "waste" when it's highly concentrated, not when the animals are managed well.

Perhaps one of the most perplexing aspects of this story is that both overgrazing (poorly managed animals) and undergrazing (or entirely removing the grazing animals) will damage grasslands. Either can lead to a downward spiral involving more bare spots in the pasture, soil compaction, and topsoil ending up in lakes, rivers, and streams as it cascades downhill with rainwater that "should" stay on-site as part of a normal, healthy rangeland.

That's not an opinion; it's a fairly noncontroversial fact within ecology. A middle-ground solution involving properly managed animals, emulating the predator-prey interaction that coevolved with these ecosystems, is the biological "sweet spot" that enhances both food production and grassland health.

We think it's interesting that meat is one of the only foods that is routinely scrutinized for concerns such as water usage and methane production.

Amid these calculations, we think it should be noted that the nutrition in grass-finished beef is far superior to rice, avocados, walnuts, and sugar. A pound of rice requires about 410 gallons of water to produce. Avocados, walnuts, and sugar have similar water requirements. Globally, 30 percent of groundwater intended for crops is used by rice, followed by wheat (12 percent), cotton (11 percent), and soybeans (3 percent).[8]

Where food is grown is quite important, and arid regions already facing water shortages may do well to rethink their crop production. These are in fact the ideal areas for holistic management.

Take almonds, for example. Almonds are tough to dislike when we're talking about flavor and nutrition, but in the US, they are one of the most water-intensive crops. The amount of blue water needed for, and gray water produced from, nut production is far greater than for typical meat production.[9] This wouldn't be of particular concern if a water-intensive crop was grown in a water-rich location, but California's Central Valley is notoriously parched. In an ironic twist, it's challenging for people living there to find adequate drinking water (there is not much to be had, and what is there is rapidly accumulating various chemical by-products of industrial agriculture), yet farmers employ the incredibly inefficient method of flood-irrigating almonds. (If you would like to learn more on this topic we recommend the film *Water and Power: A California Heist*.) California agriculture uses 80 percent of available water and only contributes 2 percent of the state's revenue. Given that two-thirds of the almonds produced in California are exported, one could make the case that California's drinking water is being exported in the form of nuts, at least in part. Although California is dry, it does receive significant rainfall at various times of the year. This fact did not escape the notice of government officials in the previous century, who stewarded a host of dams and water projects that arguably have allowed California to grow as it has, providing both electricity and a relatively stable (albeit not infinite) water supply. Although one can catch occasional news pieces suggesting that it may be time to expand the hydroelectric infrastructure of the Golden State, concerns surrounding damage to fish runs and general environmental impact will make these solutions unlikely to materialize. Now, almonds, rice, and other plant foods should play some part in our collective diets, but comparing "plant products" to "meat" is logical (and honest) only if energetic inputs, outputs, and nutritional benefits are completely considered. The irrigation of crops takes up about 70 percent of the world's freshwater withdrawals[10], but that is largely ignored in discussions of sustainability.[11]

Despite the fact that 70 percent of the planet's surface is covered in water, when we talk about water usable for drinking and good production, we are facing real challenges. Jay Famiglietti, senior water scientist at NASA Jet Propulsion Laboratory, found that two billion people across the world already rely on nonrenewable sources of water, and more than half the world's aquifers are being depleted past the "sustainability tipping point":

The irony of groundwater is that despite its critical importance to global water supplies, it attracts insufficient management attention relative to more visible surface water supplies in rivers and reservoirs. In many regions around the world, groundwater is often poorly monitored and managed. In the developing world, oversight is often non-existent.[12]

As we continue to pump water from deeper sources, the energy required to attain the water increases, and so does the price. We're currently pumping water at unsustainable rates, faster than it can naturally be replenished. Globally, agriculture accounts for almost 80 percent of water use, and at least half of this is groundwater. As we continue to drain our groundwater, many of our major rivers (the Colorado, Indus, and Yellow Rivers) no longer reach the ocean.

What we see from the industrial row-crop system consistently is compacted soil, soil and chemical runoff, and loss of topsoil. These all feed into a process that pollutes rivers, does not restore groundwater, and leaves less surface water available. This is well understood and of paramount concern. Nature "wants" to store and cycle water, and we've broken this system. The best storage of all is the tiny holes between grains of soil. When soil is degraded and compacted, these spaces are lost. Compaction also occurs when we tile and drain the soil to make it easier to farm crops. Natural ecosystems also have a more variable topography that stores water in ponds and puddles. We smooth them out to make it easier to farm—either conventionally raised animals or crops. By doing the things that make it easier to industrially farm, we enter and amplify a cycle that destroys nature's small water cycles that are vital to life.

If water is befouled, it is tough to either drink or use to grow food. The EPA considers agriculture the largest water pollution source in the United States. In industrial agriculture, synthetic chemicals and nutrients end up in our rivers and streams as runoff. This has impacts not only on the ecology of the plants, animals, and insects living in the freshwater environment but also sometimes thousands of miles away when these nutrient-enriched waters create massive "dead zones" in coastal waters because of the enhanced growth of certain aquatic organisms that, in their race to grow, consume virtually all the oxygen dissolved in these coastal waters.

Corn production uses more herbicides and insecticides and causes more runoff and water pollution than any other crop. Confined animal production also leads to water contamination, containing pathogens, antibiotics, hormones, chemicals, and heavy metals. Of all antibiotics produced in the US, 80 percent are given to livestock and poultry,[13] the majority of which (90 percent) are not sick animals—rather, the antibiotics are intended to marginally improve growth rates and prevent sickness.[14] Up to 75 percent of these antibiotics pass through the animal and into the environment unchanged.[15] Antibiotic resistance in humans is a massive public health concern, and this is exacerbated, in part, by their broad use in livestock. By contrast, when livestock are given a healthy environment and low stress, they don't need to be given preemptive antibiotics, which can dramatically cut down the incidence of antibiotic resistance.

Whether meat eaters or vegans, more people than ever are concerned about the impact their food choices have on the environment. That's a very good thing. These are important issues, but it's worth asking a few key questions about the relative merits of one's dietary choices: How much water did it take to produce your almond flour muffin, your tofurkey sandwich, and your "clean" Beyond Burger made from ultraprocessed pea protein isolate and canola? The simplistic narrative is that "plant-based" options are inherently more sustainable than meat-inclusive options. As compelling as this notion may appear on the surface, the truth of the matter might not be as cut-and-dried as we'd thought. The alternate narrative here is that beef that is raised on pasture and managed holistically could provide not only nutrient-dense protein but also a system of improved soil water capture, increased biodiversity, carbon sequestration, and long-term sustainability.

To recap, we've laid out the following arguments to the common complaints about cattle:

They emit too many greenhouse gases. Well-managed cattle can be a net carbon sink, but even in a system where there are slight emissions, the nutritional gains and the added environmental benefits of cattle (increased biodiversity, better water-holding capacity, breaking down nonnutritive foods and converting them into a nutrient-rich source of protein and fats) far outweigh the 2 percent global emissions, especially compared to other less nutritious yet higher-emission-producing foods like rice.

They're inefficient with feed. When compared with other animals, cattle actually need less "grain" because most of their lives are spent grazing on land we can't use for crops. Most of the feed cattle consume doesn't compete with human food. They can actually upcycle nutrients by converting grasses and other crop residue to protein.

They take up too much land. Not all land is usable for cropping. Cattle can graze on land we can't crop, upcycling grass to meat, a nutrient-dense food for humans. Ruminants can also be integrated into cropping systems and orchards, which increases fertility and eliminates the need for herbicides, tillage, and nitrogen, phosphorus, and potassium fertilizers. So land can be used for both livestock and crops. Once we understand that cattle can not only be made "less bad" but can be produced in a way that creates "more good," the fact that cattle production covers so much land shifts from being seen as a liability to a very material asset.

They use too much water. The methodology used to blame cattle for using water is flawed, because it includes rainwater. When looking at blue water (groundwater), even in conventional systems cattle are equal to or better than many crops like almonds, rice, avocados, walnuts, and sugar. In well-managed grazing systems, grazing animals actually improve the water-holding capacity of the soil, preventing rain from running off and driving silt into rivers.

Well-managed ruminant animals are the key to our future. We absolutely need to include them as a solution to our broken agricultural system, which has destroyed much of our soil. It's important to fully understand the nutritional gains cattle (see the previous chapter) provide to our food system in order to appreciate the environmental case. In the next chapter we'll look at the ethical case for better meat, which we feel can only be understood once a person understands the environmental argument.

We hope we have made a compelling case for why we need more ruminants grazed in the right way in order to help mitigate climate change, increase biodiversity, increase the water-holding capacity of the soil, and sequester carbon while providing nutrient-dense food. But what about the whole idea that an animal had to die for you to eat? Can't we just have these animals grazing on pasture and allow them to live out their lives to an old age without having to slaughter them for food? These questions and more will be addressed in the next section.

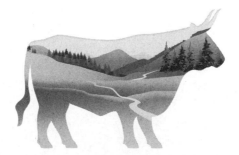

PART III

THE ETHICAL CASE FOR (BETTER) MEAT

CHAPTER 13

IS EATING ANIMALS IMMORAL?

The first sections of this book are arguably more "objective" in character. If we talk about optimum nutrition, for example, we *can* define what that is in fairly concrete terms, lean on concepts such as nutrient density and the relative satiety food offers, and then compare and contrast various dietary interventions.

Ethics is tougher to objectively pin down.

For example, one could make the case—and we will—that eating a diet built from grazing animals, fruits, vegetables, and roots and tubers is not only more nutrient dense (healthier) but arguably more ethical because it is more environmentally sustainable. And what if we consider that a properly managed food system—one that relies on regenerative food production strategies—is not only sustainable, and healthy, but also reduces death and suffering? Couldn't that be a way of causing "least harm"?

These arguments may be tough for some to hear. One might raise the objection that it's not the total number but the intent. How can one possibly raise an animal knowing it will be eaten? How can you justify intentionally killing another animal for you to live?

When dealing with such thorny issues, it's easy to reach an impasse. Still, we feel there is common ground to be established between ethically motivated nonmeat eaters and those who argue for better meat. Desiring to cause least harm through your food choices is a noble ambition. We completely respect one's religious or personal choice not to eat meat. If some people don't like the taste or have a hard time with the idea of eating meat, that's totally OK. We both have some very good friends who avoid meat, even though they know that this is not an environmentally better or healthier choice. However, there are some people who feel it's morally superior to avoid meat and would like everyone to adopt a plant-based diet. The following perhaps encapsulates our point; Joel Salatin, founder of Polyface Farms had this to say on the topic: "If vegans will let me raise the food I want to feed my family, I will be sure to raise enough of the food they want to feed their families." When considering ethics and morality, this is an interesting point to consider. Joel and many people like him are not interested in converting anyone to their way of living; they are more than happy to help facilitate a way of life different from their own. But this generous sentiment is all too often *not* reciprocated by vegan-backed media, academia, and social platforms. Their stated goal is to make meat consumption and production illegal, or inaccessible. The CEO of vegan company Impossible Burger, Pat Brown, has said, "The primary goal is to effectively eliminate the use of animals in the food system."[1]

In this section, we'd like to challenge the logic that some use to justify that position. When someone argues that all meat is "evil," decentralized, regional, and regenerative food systems, which offer both better quality of life for animals and more sustainable food for humans, are excluded from the discussion. From a globalization perspective, this is also a challenging ethical position as the folks making the case to remove all animal inputs in the global food system are pushing for food policies that would destroy the food systems in developing countries. Is it in fact "ethical" for a largely white, wealthy, Western vegan-centric elite to dictate what constitutes proper morality for every human (and nonhuman) on the planet?

Our position is that even those who avoid eating meat should fight for all farmed animals to have good lives and humane deaths. There are legitimate animal welfare concerns with how some producers and slaughterhouses handle farmed animals. At the same time, one must question how eliminating meat from your plate and only eating plants can really be the most ethical choice when we consider the industrial, synthetic chemical row-crop-centric model that entails. In order to have a truly educated debate on the ethics of eating animals, one must have a very deep understanding of food production. As we argued in the environmental section, in order to have a truly regenerative food system, we must include animals one way or the other. We also illustrated in the nutrition chapter that animals provide critical nutrients that humans need to thrive. We will now advance the argument that eating these animals is the logical continuation of this thread of reasoning and that eating well-raised animals is the most ethical diet.

TAKE A DEEP BREATH . . .

Let's put our emotions to the side for a moment and acknowledge that animals are an integral part of a regenerative farming system, that death is an inescapable truth of nature, and that meat provides nutrient-dense food for humans.

It's widely known that appeals to emotions are quite persuasive and can have a greater effect on our decision-making than logical arguments. When presented with gruesome antimeat images and language designed to evoke guilt, fear, anxiety, pity, anger, sadness, or disgust, people are often won over. Reality is sometimes counterintuitive. Not all farmed animals are raised by people wishing to inflict pain, and not all slaughterhouses abuse and torture the animals. And not all death is "bad."

Perhaps the most pressing problem for sustainability, regardless of whether we are discussing the potential role of animals in a food system or appropriate measures to address climate change, is that the vast majority of Westernized populations have become divorced from nature. We see nature as a place to visit, not a system we are a part of. Because of this, many people simply can't come to grips with the idea that death is inevitable, unavoidable, and important for new life. Many think any death is wrong. We can sympathize with this position and understand why people feel this way. Death is scary, so why inflict it on another animal if we don't need to?

OUR FEAR OF DEATH

Until recently in our history, death was something we dealt with on a regular basis. For most of human history we cared for dying family members in our homes, but now we send them to nursing homes and hospice care. Today, our experience with the death of humans is mainly through images we see in horror films or video games. If you've ever been at the bedside of a loved one who was suffering, you know how awful the dying process can be. Most doctors and nurses are familiar with how many family members want to keep someone alive, even when the person dying just wants to go. It's a really painful situation to watch. We're also terrified of our own deaths. Books on longevity, serums to keep us youthful, and diets promising us that we can live forever are bestsellers. We seek to avoid old age and death at all costs. We don't want to see it, think about it, or face the fact that we will die. (More than half of Americans don't have a will.)[2] We just don't want to accept that our days are numbered. But folks, the sad truth is that none of us is making it out of here alive.

When it comes to food and the animals we eat, most families used to slaughter and process their own livestock. Before our gigantic shift in food production, beef was grass-fed and pigs and chickens were raised in backyards. Killing an animal for meat was necessary, done with respect, and the entire animal was used.

Today, the killing of animals for meat no longer happens near our homes or in cities and is often considered dirty lowbrow work; we've "farmed" that job out to slaughterhouses. Most of us are entirely removed from how our food is produced. Most people have never hunted, fished, or processed an animal. Butcher shops once proudly displayed pigs' heads in their cases and full duck bodies in the window, but they can now (at least in the US) generally only show the boneless, skinless, plastic-wrapped parts. People don't want to acknowledge that their steak came from an actual animal and don't want to know how its life ended. While many watch nature programs about lions or snakes taking down their prey, we would never show a human processing a farm animal in a slaughterhouse (except in alarming antimeat propaganda films). We may enjoy bucolic depictions of ranchers herding cattle, but those who eat meat usually don't want to know that these animals were killed.

But taking an animal from a living, breathing, eating being to the next phase of its existence—feeding people—isn't necessarily gruesome, and it can actually be remarkably spiritual. In order to fully appreciate the importance of this process, we need to recognize that all life has to end in order for new life to begin. Animals can either die in the wild (which is seldom "humane") or we, as humans, can take care to ensure a low-stress process. As opposed to coyotes, people can treat the animals we eat in a way that arguably minimizes suffering.

Contrary to the prejudices of many vegans, responsible producers really do care about how their animals have lived and how they will die. It's important to them that the animals they've cared for are given respectful treatment in their last hours. This is why Diana is on the board of Animal Welfare Approved, an organization helping to improve living conditions and ensuring humane handling techniques at slaughterhouses.

We have made this point previously, but it is worth repeating: reducing this story to a false dichotomy, one that insists the only moral way forward is eating *no* meat, virtually ensures that the worst practices and most suffering of animals will continue. It can be easy to think that avoiding all meat is the *only* ethical choice we can make. But we are all part of a food web and the inevitable cycle of life, which includes death.

Once one has a full understanding of regenerative agriculture, then most quickly realize that avoiding animal consumption altogether does little to change our system. We need nutrients to grow our kale, which we can either get from mining and petroleum or from animal inputs. If more people knew how food is produced, there would be fewer arguments about whether animals are important. In a stroke of irony that would be humorous were it not so tragic, when people give up grazing animals and shift more to eating factory-raised chicken and meatless burger patties, they're actually propping up a system that is destroying our topsoil and, ultimately, ending more lives.

WHAT DOES NATURAL DEATH LOOK LIKE?

Once people understand that animals are an important part of the nutrient cycle, the following questions often come up: If we need animals for soil health, why can't we just let them graze to sequester carbon and die a natural death? Why is it necessary to eat them?

Because many of us are not familiar with the death process, it's easy to idealize natural death. But the problem is, most animals (just like most people) don't just die peacefully in their sleep. There are many ways animals die "naturally." From being hunted by a coyote or lion to having a broken leg and being slowly picked off alive by hyenas and vultures, natural death is rarely pretty. We thought we'd illustrate this point with a story about Diana's daughter.

IT'S IMPOSSIBLE TO BE VEGAN: LESSONS FROM A TEN-YEAR-OLD GIRL

We have a sweet little pond on the farm where my kids enjoy catching frogs and going fishing. They spend hours down there and find all sorts of creatures, make up games, and do other kid things.

One morning during spring break, my daughter, Phoebe, and her friend went down to the pond, buckets in hand to catch some creatures. They were horrified to find a dead sheep. They came running into the kitchen where I was cooking lunch for the farm crew and insisted I come see it. As we walked out toward the pond, they vividly described how "intestines were all over the grass, the heart was near a rock, and there was an explosion of blood everywhere." When we finally got to the scene, I had to agree with their depiction. The carcass had been completely gutted, and the organs were gone. There was a lot of blood and wool all over the grass. There were flies everywhere. It was really gross.

"Looks like a coyote got to this one," I said. "These things happen on a farm sometimes. We do our best to protect them with fencing and the dogs, but sometimes the coyotes figure it out." The two girls were quiet as we walked back to the house for lunch. I thought to myself that this might be one of those traumatic scenes from childhood that sticks with them unless I somehow defuse it. "Um, does anybody need to talk about this? Are you guys feeling OK about what you saw?"

"It was the grossest thing I've ever seen!" said my daughter's friend. My daughter just kept her head down and didn't say much.

After lunch, I was sitting at my computer working. The girls were playing when I heard Phoebe say to her friend, "Hang on, I have to go tell my mom something." She came running to me and hugged me and broke down crying. I can only imagine being a ten-year-old girl, happily looking forward to catching some good frogs, and being jolted by that carnage.

"It's totally normal for you to have been surprised by what you saw. Nature can be pretty cruel sometimes. This is how things often die in nature. When we raise animals here on the farm, we try to make sure they die in the least stressful way possible. When they get processed, it's quick. Out in the real world, when a prey animal dies, it can be pretty drawn out and painful. Coyotes need to eat, too."

Now I had to drop off Phoebe's friend and tell the mom what the girls saw and hope that she wouldn't sue me. Luckily, the mom is a member of the farm CSA (community-supported agriculture) and has copies of my books, so I was relieved when she wasn't furious with me. I felt really bad for what her daughter had seen. Not many suburban kids have experiences like that on playdates. Phew!

That evening, when my husband and I were tucking in Phoebe for bed, she started crying again. She needed to further process what she saw. I was glad Andrew was there with me. He's an incredible dad and does a great job explaining complicated things in an easy way to the kids. (Most kids think he's a superhero.) He told Phoebe how the sheep lived a good life, had fed the coyote, and how he buried the rest of the sheep's body in the compost and it's going into the soil to feed the vegetables.

"Soil is a living thing. There are tiny organisms in the soil that need the nutrients in that sheep. Those bones in the sheep will turn into calcium to grow better kale. Everything dies and comes back again," he said.

Phoebe sat right up. "Wait a minute, you're telling me that those bones turn into vegetables? Can you *taste* them? I'm eating *bones* when I eat vegetables?"

"No, you can't taste them, but you are eating bones and blood and lots of other things when you eat vegetables," he explained.

"So then it's impossible to be a vegan! If the soil is living, and everything dead comes back to life, then you can't possibly eat without eating something that has died." she exclaimed.

I have to say I was thrilled at how quickly those little wheels in her brain cranked. The kid is sharp and made a leap quickly that helped her process what she saw. She slept without any nightmares of sheep blood. She hasn't brought it up since. The subject is closed for now. She gets it, and she got the big picture on her own without me having to make all the associations for her. I wish all kids (and adults) had the chance to learn about life and death by roaming freely outside.

If our goal is to end needless suffering, let's consider more "humane" ways we humans can end life instead of leaving it up to the hands of "nature." In nature, most animals are killed by another animal to be eaten. This usually involves a stressful encounter with a stronger animal possessing big teeth, and a drawn-out and painful death. It's true that the most commonly killed animals in nature are the old or sick, but that's simply because those are the easiest ones to catch. If the lion had its way, it would certainly choose the biggest zebra it could find. Is it wrong for humans to take the lives of strong, healthy animals? Should we only eat sick and older animals? On the other hand, one could argue that humans taking the lives of animals in their prime limits their suffering because they don't have a chance to suffer from a broken leg or a debilitating illness in old age.

As opposed to animals in the wild, humans have the ability to be the most compassionate killers on the planet. Compare slowly, painfully dying in "nature" to being quickly rendered unconscious followed by a slit to the throat. Slaughterhouses that employ humane handling techniques do their best to make sure the animal dies quickly and with the least stress and pain possible. Most people working there do honestly care about this process and take pride in taking the animal to the next phase of its existence—feeding lots of people. By contrast, hyenas are not very "humane" when it comes to their treatment of wildebeests, often eating them while they're still alive.

As illustrated in Diana's story, sheep are sometimes attacked and eaten by coyotes. Farmers do their best to protect them, but sometimes it happens. Many animal activists will say farmers are simply protecting their financial investment, but we can tell you that it's also upsetting to see an animal you're responsible for hurt. But consider this: Is eating a sheep wrong of the coyote? Does this sheep have rights? If so, did the coyote violate the sheep's rights by eating it? Coyotes play an important role in nature, and they need to eat, too! What about the eagles and hawks that eat farm chickens, or eat field mice, or rabbits, or your cat? If a hawk eats your cat, but minutes before, your cat ate a mouse, which animal is "worse"? And by owning the cat, was the mouse's death partly your fault? Who is violating whom? Who decides who gets to eat and who does not? Who decides which animal is more important than the other?

These are difficult questions, questions that rarely have clean, unambiguous answers. This is perhaps one of the most troubling things about folks who insist on the mantra "No meat, no matter what." How does one arrive at this degree of certitude on such a remarkably complex topic?

Besides violent death, disease may take over an animal and kill it. This process is also not painless. But let's say the animal is completely protected from predators, doesn't die from sickness or infection, and lives to a very old age. By the end of its life, its organs start to fail and the animal can no longer eat or drink. Maybe it goes blind or breaks a leg. Is this process painless and fast? Is it "humane"?

Is it better to allow an animal to suffer at the hands of another predator than ensure a humane death? Life is great when you're young and healthy, but nobody stays young and healthy forever. As caregivers, responsible farmers ensure that their animals are well fed, have access to clean water, are treated for infections, and enjoy a relatively stress-free life. This is much more comfortable than life in the wild, where food can be scarce, cuts can become deadly infections, and there's no fencing to protect them from predators.

We've all seen nature shows with herds of healthy-looking zebras or deer in the wild, but the reality is that they are only healthy because the sick and old have been culled (eaten and removed from the herd), and their numbers kept in check by predators. Populations need to be controlled in some way. Do we, as humans, need to remove the predators? Would that be more humane?

British philosopher David Pearce sees the natural world as a terrible place begging for the hand of man to set it right. He sees predatory animals as victimizing their prey, and the scales of justice may only be set right once *all* predators have either been eliminated or genetically and neurologically reprogrammed to no longer eat other animals. Although his position has not garnered wide support, it illustrates that even the most highly educated among us have become so divorced from the natural world and so afraid of "suffering" that we can be tempted to seriously propose the end of life on earth just to avoid it.[3] It is like a real-life incarnation of Thanos, the archvillain from the Marvel Comics universe, who considers the only way of "saving" life is by exterminating half of all living beings.

The above point is worth expanding on. In an effort to "save the planet" and "end suffering" the antimeat worldview in fact guarantees a loss of species diversity and leans on a system that has an expiration date in the near future. This is a remarkable amount of psycho-emotional gymnastics that, while (possibly) well intentioned, is a medicine worse than the disease.

But even if we grant that animals are a vital part of agriculture, why do we need to eat them? So, we should use animals to produce better soil . . . but just let them live out their lives and die naturally? As we've seen, a "natural death" is difficult to define, and as people who raise animals in this way have learned, waiting for the natural process of death to take an animal can be nothing short of heart wrenching. Some might even call *that* process unethical, if not positively cruel. If you want kale, you should be open to the notion that animals should play a role in the food system, and that we may need to eat more animals, not fewer. This scenario means we will maximally capture solar energy in the form of plants, and the animals convert that energy into good soil, fertilizer for other plants, *and* healthy nutrients for people—in a word, life.

We recognize that this is already a long and technical book, but physicist Jeremy England makes an important point in a recent paper. He argues that the purpose of life is to enhance entropy, or the relative disorder in the world or universe.[4] This may be an unsatisfying case for the more spiritually minded, but it has profound implications regardless of one's religious stance. In the short term, life works against entropy by harnessing the energy around us (mainly from the sun, although a few systems on the ocean floor exist largely independent from this system) and creating *more* life. This is called a nonequilibrium process (or nonequilibrium thermodynamics, for the technically inclined), and this concept makes the case that we'd do well to foster as much of this nonequilibrium process as we can. What does this mean in practical terms? Encourage as many plants as possible to harness as much sunlight as possible. Have as many animals as possible consuming both plants and animals. Encourage this system to be as diversified and resilient as possible. In short, this looks like a lot of grass and grazing animals; it does *not* look like row crops as far as the eye can see, all dependent on unsustainable synthetic chemical inputs. If we pause for a moment and imagine an earth without humans, or the earth before humans, both these scenarios involve a remarkable amount of life. And death.

Perhaps if humans had a more conscious sense of our own mortality (to say nothing of an appreciation for our place in nature) and understood how sustainable food production really worked, we wouldn't be so afraid of the death process and we'd do more to ensure humane death for both humans and farm animals.

SENTIENCE

There was an interesting story floating around the web a while back about an octopus in zoo who was able to squeeze out a tube, scoot across the floor, and slither down a pipe, presumably out to the ocean.[5] Think *Finding Nemo*. There are even videos of an octopus taking photos of the people watching it.[6] What likely makes these stories and images go viral is that folks are blown away by how smart the animals are. But what about other animals? Are they less or more brilliant or worthy of not being eaten than an octopus? Who decides if they're "better" or "worse" than a chicken or a bison? Possibly what was so intriguing and compelling to folks about this video was how they could *relate* to the octopus. The octopus was smart, but only according to what humans consider smart. What about all the other animals in the world that do very clever things?

This is an interesting conundrum. On the one hand, some in the antimeat scene suggest that humanity is a blight unto the earth, yet these same people make the case that the more like "us" an organism is (sentience), the more unethical it is to eat it. Plants, they argue, do not respond like humans or animals do to "pain," so it is ethically acceptable to eat them. But there's a fallacy lurking in this position, since plants do in fact respond to attempts to eat them, via chemical warfare and warning neighbors. Trees can "talk" below ground through fungal networks.[7] They can direct nutrients to other trees, know which trees are kin and which are not, and can even "feed" dying trees in an effort to keep them alive.[8] When a tree is being eaten by a certain pest, that tree can turn on chemicals that will make its leaves taste bitter. It can also alert other trees that this pest is nearby, making those trees taste bitter, too. It can even send out a call message to beneficial insects that will eat the pest.[9] Other plants have been documented "reaching" for sounds, and it's common knowledge they move toward light. Peas will grow in the direction of a trellis, even if it's not directly above them. Plants, it turns out, are indeed "feelers" and "communicators."[10] Because they don't have eyes to see, does that make a tree less important than a rabbit? What about worms? Are worms less important or more important than kale? Is a small fish or a fruit fly's life more worthy of saving than a three-hundred-year-old maple tree?

Let's think about other animals. What about bees? We couldn't live at all without these and other pollinators, yet only a small group is advocating to get rid of pesticides. Let's be clear on this point: the monocrop food production system "works" only to the degree that synthetic fertilizers, pesticides, herbicides, and fungicides are available and effective. This very system is destroying pollinator populations and degrading topsoil.

And is it possible that there are animals that are special and important and valuable that aren't similar to humans? Is it possible that we might not know everything about what makes other species "intelligent" or "important"? What makes one food OK to eat and another food not OK? Are other humans only valuable to you if they're similar to you? The enlightened knee-jerk reaction is "Oh, everyone matters!" This is all oddly reminiscent of *Animal Farm*: some animals certainly are more equal than others.

LEAST HARM

We've touched a bit on the idea of doing the least harm several times so far. Many people will readily agree that the goal for all of us should be to cause the least harm to the natural world through our lifestyle practices. Human activity can be incredibly destructive, and those who attempt to reduce their impact through their food choices should be applauded. However, regardless of one's good intentions, avoiding meat is not ultimately consistent with a food system generating the "least harm."

Environmentally and for animal welfare reasons, grass-fed beef is a far better choice than industrially raised chicken. One could argue that even typical beef is better than industrially raised chicken. As we made clear in the environment section, you can get nearly five hundred pounds from one beef steer. How many chickens would you need for that much meat? Industrially raised chickens eat 100 percent grain (grown on land we could be using for human food) and live 100 percent of their lives indoors. Even "cage-free" chickens live indoors. Unless your chicken is pasture raised, it's probably spent most or all its life indoors. Did you know that there are also no humane handling laws for chicken slaughter? Similarly, pescatarians might be shocked to learn that there are no humane handling laws for how fish die. Even cattle that end up on feedlots are outdoors, can move freely, and are legally subject to humane handling at slaughter. The same can't be said for CAFO chicken or fish (wild or farmed). The message "stop eating all meat" isn't convincing folks and does nothing to change these poor practices. It diverts energy and resources into fundamentally unsustainable endeavors such as CAFO chicken, farmed fish, and lab-grown meat.

As we've explored in the environmental section, when we make room for a field of crops, we destroy habitat (killing things in the process), and indirectly, when we annihilate an animal's food source to make way for more soy fields, we kill the native animals. If we eliminate animals from pastureland, we'll destroy that land, too. And if we just allow the ruminants to "live out their lives and die a natural death" without managing their numbers, then either they will consume all the food and die or the wolves get to eat and we're stuck with corn and soy.

Let's look at the actual process of farming vegetables and grains. First, the farmer tills the soil, killing worms, mice, and any other animals that have made a home there over the winter months. During the growing of the crops, pesticides kill insects and poison the animals that eat them. Then there's the exposed soil and runoff of these chemicals that lands in local rivers and streams, killing fish and other aquatic life. When it comes time to harvest, the tractors kill any small mammals like rabbits that are in the way. Even organic farmers kill pests on their farms; they just do it differently than conventional farmers—namely, through beneficial insects, organic pesticides, and with guns or traps. We also have to consider the deaths to predation of exposing animals that once had a natural ecosystem cover. Are those who eat crops responsible for the death of a rabbit who can no longer hide from the hawk? Billions of animals are also killed around our granaries and other food storage facilities, restaurants, and cities, which, if it didn't happen, could assure our starvation.

Animal death is a by-product of plant production. It's inescapable.

There have been several attempts to calculate how many critters die in field harvest.[11] How many deaths are you causing per calorie you eat? At forty rodent deaths per acre, and six million calories per acre of wheat, that's 150,000 calories per rodent life. Let's be generous and assume only one head of cattle per acre yields approximately five hundred pounds of beef. At approximately 1,100 calories per pound, that's 550,000 calories per cow life! So perhaps, if you want to save more animal lives, eat beef, not wheat.

Not to mention, beef is far more nutritious than wheat. The difference would be even more astounding if we looked at deaths per nutrient.

Another person to question whether avoiding meat is consistent with the principle of least harm is Stephen Davis from the Department of Animal Sciences at Oregon State University. When considering the mortality rate of every opossum, sparrow, starling, rat, mouse, partridge, turkey, rabbit, vole, and the many species of amphibians that die through plowing, disking, harrowing, cultivating, and through the chemicals used to kill insects and weeds, one can clearly see that one large ruminant (like a cow) on a diet of grass is causing much less harm than a diet rich in field crops.

Also, as you'll remember from the environmental section, well-managed cattle increase wildlife populations, improve ecosystem health, increase the water-holding capacity of the soil (making rainfall less likely to run off), and sequester carbon. There are no monocrop fields of irrigated and chemically sprayed soy in nature. We have done this to the native grasslands and forests that once were there, and in the process we have eliminated the natural habitat for all the living creatures that once lived there.

Some folks call for a "rewilding" of our grasslands and for humans just to use arable land for crop production. This sounds like a great solution . . . until you realize that wild animals need predators in order to keep their populations in check. Because humans have not only reduced the populations of wild ruminants like bison, deer, and elk but also their natural predators, we're seeing huge issues with overpopulation and overgrazing. This is particularly an issue in the Northeast. Deer are eating people's gardens and farmer's crops (an open salad bar!), but many communities don't want hunters to help manage the problem. Deer are also overeating forest underbrush, which forms a critical habitat for birds, in addition to causing car accidents and leading to many tragic human deaths. The solution is either to bring back predators like wolves in large numbers to manage the wildlife populations in suburbia (and displace a lot of humans) or to hunt them. The truth is, most hunters are dedicated conservationists.

Let's look at another example. Is almond milk causing less harm than cow milk? Nut milks are certainly staples of many meat-free kitchens. California produces 80 percent of the world's almonds, yet most are exported to China. In essence, we are exporting our water and nutrients to another country. When we build dams and divert rivers to irrigate water-intensive crops that are produced in deserts, fish lose their lives, and the animals and plants that need those fish also die. Yes, many trees thrive on the nutrients from fish. In some parts of California, local residents even have no drinking water because large corporations continue to irrigate almonds and other crops.

What about palm oil, which is commonly used in processed foods and sold in health food stores? Is palm oil vegan? The World Wildlife Fund estimates that an area equivalent to three hundred football fields of rainforest is cleared each hour to make space for the production of palm oil, endangering habitat for orangutans and Sumatran tigers. Videos on the internet highlight the impact on orangutans, but what about the human impact of this industry? Children often carry heavy loads of palm fruit, suffering from injuries and heat exhaustion, for little or no pay. Somehow the human element doesn't make the headlines, but the orangutans do.

Have you ever spent a day harvesting vegetables? It can be hot, backbreaking, and incredibly dangerous work. Do you know if your tomatoes were picked by an exploited immigrant or child? Do you know if the workers were paid a fair wage? The Association of Farmworker Opportunity Programs estimates that of the over two hundred million children working worldwide, 70 percent of them work in agriculture, and there are between four hundred thousand and five hundred thousand child farmworkers in the United States. Many of the laws that protect child labor don't apply to agriculture.[12] Should human suffering for our produce be considered when looking at a diet that causes least harm?

What about chocolate? If you're not buying fair-trade chocolate, then it's quite possible you're indirectly participating in human trafficking, kidnapping, and child labor. Most of the major brands sold in the US and Europe source their chocolate from places where these practices are prevalent.[13] Over two million children are illegally harvesting chocolate in western Africa. Once considered host to the most biodiverse animal populations in Africa, today the Ivory Coast has converted 90 percent of its protected land to chocolate production, which has had a devastating effect on wildlife populations. And while we don't hear this in the news, one chocolate bar made from deforestation generates the same carbon emissions as driving 4.9 miles in a car.[14] And how about bananas, America's number one (or two, depending on the year) fruit? When aerial spraying of cancerous chemicals lands on local homes and schools to bring us our cheap food, causing illness, birth defects, and death, is that food still vegan? Are we only concerned with animal lives, or do human lives count?

How much energy and water is required to produce, package, transport, and store this meatless alternative? What is the expense of this energy? Was the factory powered by natural gas from fracking or solar energy? Was it transported using oil? Entire wars have been fought over oil, and many human lives have been lost. Perhaps the principle of least harm could also include less processing, less energy, more local, more whole food?

Historically, humans in northern climates relied on animals for fats, and also for fertilizer. But when you start to think about how one might consume a 100 percent plant-based diet in a northern or hot and arid climate, all sorts of questions emerge. How will you grow the fats? Most vegans in North America get their fats from coconuts, palm, or avocados. Canola (also called rape plant) grows in the north, but requires a lot of land to grow and lots of energy to extract. "Green manure" can be grown to enhance soil quality, but that also requires tillable land that can be used to grow crops. And flat tillable land is at a premium. Perhaps in a warm humid climate, like the Caribbean, a diet without animal fats is more feasible for humans, but if you're looking to grow vegetables, you'll still need to clear rainforest or dramatically improve the poor soil of many of the islands. And what about in arid regions? Is it truly ethical to suggest that a plant-based diet is optimal to people who don't have the water to spare to irrigate almonds? Milk, raw meat, blood, and honey are the traditional food of the Maasai of Kenya and northern Tanzania. They eat few to no vegetables. In fact, two-thirds of their diet comes from animal fats (yet they have low rates of heart disease). Do we tell them now that they must eat more whole grains and kale? Is it ethical to impose our plant-based morals on this already healthy population, where vegetables don't grow well? If it is not moral to wag one's finger at these populations and force them to abandon their traditional diets, why is it ethical to do so in Westernized society?

At the end of the day, blood is spilled, and lots of harm is caused in the production of produce. It's impossible to limit the idea of least harm to flesh on the plate. If you know that your actions will cause death as a side effect, and you still do it, then you are causing death. If you didn't intend to kill something, but something is killed as a known side effect of your actions, does this somehow make it OK? Let's consider a hypothetical scenario. If you drive to a certain store to buy some tofu and accidentally run over a chipmunk on the way, did you still kill it? Yes. But do you have any guilt or culpability? Maybe not. It is clear that you had neither foreknowledge nor intention that your driving would kill the chipmunk. But what if you knew, for a fact, that each time you went to that store to buy tofu, you were definitely going to run over an entire family of chipmunks on your way. If you know that you are going to kill the chipmunks on the way to the store to buy tofu, is it still morally OK to go to the store, even if you're not *intending* to kill the chipmunks?

If you're aware that your actions cause a known effect, then intent is present.

If you value the lives of rabbits or chipmunks as much as that of a cow, and are truly looking to kill the least amount of lives to feed your own, then we propose that killing one well-raised cow that lived on pasture is actually causing less death than the number of animal lives that are lost by modern row-cropping techniques. In the last analysis, the principle of least harm may actually require the consumption of large herbivores (red meat).[15]

CHAPTER 14

WHY DID MEAT BECOME TABOO?

We all need a sense of belonging and meaning in life. Having a tribe gives us a much-needed feeling of community. We all want to feel part of a group of people with similar beliefs. For some, religion is the path. For others, it's a community-centered gym. This is arguably why the CrossFit movement became so popular. Being part of a group of people that all believe that meat is the wrong answer is another sort of tribe.

Throughout history, many religions have had some set of food rules. Although beyond the scope of this book, there are some fascinating (and very long) books on the religious history of vegetarianism. While there are many religions that restrict certain meats or refuse meat altogether, it's probable that these customs originated for sanitary reasons. Back in the days before we understood germ theory, old meat really *was* dirty because of the lack of refrigeration, and avoiding it made some sense. Many religions that believe in reincarnation feel that it's not OK to eat an animal, as it could be your grandmother.

The Bible tells us that humans have been given dominion over animals (Genesis 1:26) and after the flood, "Every moving thing that lives shall be food for you" (Genesis 9:3). "For one believes that he may eat all things: another, who is weak, eats herbs" (Romans 14:2). However, others believed that because permission for meat-eating was granted after the fall of sin, vegetarianism is the "pure" state we should once again return to. In medieval Europe, however, refusing to eat meat was seen as a sign that one may also worship the devil. This led to a declaration in 1215 that communion wafers were the *literal* flesh of Christ, in an effort to separate out the true believers from the vegetarian heretics.[1]

Today, meat has become symbolic of murder, power, dominance, gluttony, and Western wealth. Many idealize vegetarians as not only healthier but also more enlightened, civilized, pure, and righteous. In a certain sense, veganism and vegetarianism have become religions unto themselves. Where you shop for food and what items end up in your cart says a lot about your ethics in today's society. Avoiding meat is often a choice that's much less about health and the environment than it is about proving one's political and ethical sophistication. Meat eaters are often viewed as backward. How can you possibly care about animals if you eat them? How can you possibly be against nuclear war or pro women's rights if you eat meat? Is it possible to be a *good person* if you eat meat?

When it comes to the "morality" of any given diet, some might imagine a hierarchy like this:

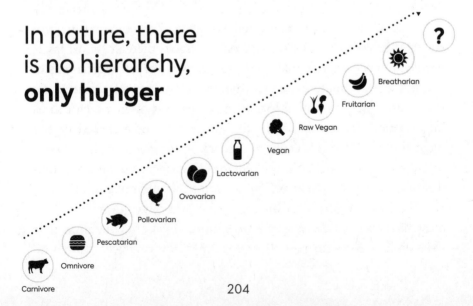

In nature, there is no hierarchy, only hunger

Breatharian
?
Fruitarian
Raw Vegan
Vegan
Lactovarian
Ovovarian
Pollovarian
Pescatarian
Omnivore
Carnivore

Many people classify the "enlightened-ness" of a diet according to how much and what type of animals and plants one consumes. It's just assumed that cattle are worse than chickens, but why is this? How is eating a fish better than an elk? How are eggs (the unborn embryos of a chicken) "cleaner" to eat than chicken flesh? Death certainly does happen in the egg business. What do you think happens to those little baby male chicks? What about cheese, is this better to eat than killing a cow? What happens to those male cows in the dairy industry? By eating cheese, one supports the veal industry, and this means supporting death. Vegetarians can only exist if there are meat eaters to consume the by-products of their diet. Eating bread entails being comfortable with all the mice that are poisoned at the granary.

The vilification of beef and fawning over chicken is particularly troublesome. One must wonder why cattle are deemed so karmically worse than chicken as a food source to so many people. Is it just the lies we've been told about how unhealthy beef is, or maybe because we're told that they're so bad for the environment? Is it because cows seem to have more "feelings," since with their big brown eyes it's easy to think of them as pets? Are chicken and seafood "cleaner" because the flesh is white and doesn't look bloody? The portions are small and can fit in your hand, and rarely are sold with bones to remind us of their animal origins.

The idea of chicken being "cleaner" than red meat is remarkably ill informed, as you're much more likely to get sick from a foodborne pathogen by eating chicken than by eating beef. Chicken are most associated with salmonella. Annually, salmonella causes 1.2 million illnesses, 23,000 hospitalizations, and 450 deaths.[2] In contrast, the main issue in the beef supply is *E. coli*, which causes an estimated 96,000 illnesses, 3,200 hospitalizations and 31 deaths in the US each year.[3] Absent an understanding of natural systems, it may be confusing why this is the case, but simply put, grazing animals are well suited to living in large groups; chickens are not. Both authors have raised chickens and can tell you that they are far from clean animals. Could it be that people often see boneless skinless chicken breast like tofu—a pale piece of protein?

Then we move up on the food-as-spirituality ladder to those who choose not to eat any animal protein at all. Are all animals more important than plants? Does one's "intention" absolve one of the blood inherent in all food production? Plants are indeed sentient,[4] but even if you don't consider them "equal" to animals, plants also consume other living things like worms, beetles, bees, and bacteria in order to survive. What about plants that are grown in a monocrop system? Chemicals poison birds and butterflies, rabbits and mice are run over by tractors, and vast fields of monocrop vegetables displace native populations of animals that once lived on the land. Even the cultivation of kale causes death, whether it's grown by synthetic fertilizer or even organically. In the case of chemical agriculture, the soil is the primary victim, with "everything else" being collateral damage. The farming of vegetables is not humane to rabbits. Even in an organic system, there is animal death. Is death

FARMING IMPACTS ON BIODIVERSITY

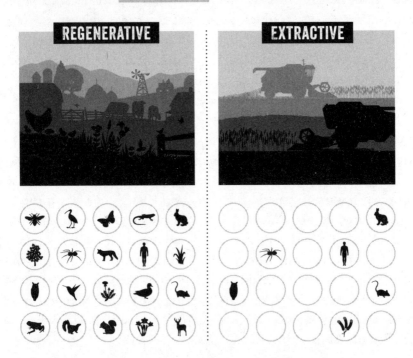

REGENERATIVE   EXTRACTIVE

less harmful to an animal if you don't intend it? Shall we strive for a diet of least intended harm or less actual harm? This is where the simple narrative of "plants good, meat bad" falls apart. How the food is produced is far more important than what the food is.

What is perhaps most fascinating and potentially dangerous about the plant-based hierarchy is that the closer you get to the top, the further you remove biodiversity and the further you remove yourself from nature. Is being a breatharian really nirvana? Breatharians assert that if you're pure enough, you don't need plants or animals to survive—you can just absorb the energy from sunlight into your being.

A major criticism of many Western societies is that it's hierarchical, but if we treat food as a test of our purity, how are we not creating yet another hierarchy? Does this show a deep understanding of the many differences in the world? In nature, there is no hierarchy, only hunger; we are not living in a pyramid, we live in a web. Humans are only one part of the web, depending on all others in the web to survive. We need the bees, the birds, the snakes, the fish, the grasslands, the rivers. We need as much diversity as possible in order to thrive. Our industrial food system eliminates biodiversity. A diet that eliminates animals relies on a food system that is wholly dependent upon industrial agricultural processes.

Not only is diet perhaps wrongly entangled with morality but modern-day vegetarianism is entangled with religious groups in ways that you might not have known. One of the most influential religious groups to condemn meat in the Western world is the Seventh-Day Adventist Church (SDA). You may remember we mentioned this group in chapter four in our analysis of prominent nutrition research. While the church officially formed in 1863, Seventh-Day Adventism began as a distinct movement nearly twenty years earlier following the so-called Great Disappointment of the Millerite movement when Christ failed to return to earth on October 22, 1844. At seventeen Ellen G. Harmon (White), had a vision that explained that event away. Cofounder of the Seventh-Day Adventist Church, Harmon experienced over two thousand dreams and visions in her life time, as the Lord's messenger sharing the spirit of prophecy. Ellen G. White's health reform vision of 1863 was the beginning of her antimeat messaging. She claimed the Garden of Eden diet was the God-given diet for man and that meat was a toxic stimulant as bad as, if not worse than alcohol or tobacco:

Meat is not essential for health or strength, else the Lord made a mistake when He provided for Adam and Eve before their fall . . . Flesh food has a tendency to animalize the nature, to rob men and women of that love and sympathy which they should feel for every one, and to give the lower passions control over the higher powers of being. If meat-eating were ever healthful, it is not safe now. Cancers, tumors, pulmonary diseases are largely caused by meat-eating.[5]

Having worked for Ellen G. White since he was just twelve years old, John Harvey Kellogg also believed that eating meat led to masturbation—considered then one of the most serious sins.[*] Kellogg's Corn Flakes were invented at Battle Creek Sanitarium in 1894, along with the first meat analogues, Nuttose and Protose.

Sylvester Graham preceded John Harvey Kellogg as an itinerant preacher and health reformer in the 1830s. He equated eating meat with impure thoughts, and his followers are credited with inventing graham flour and crackers. Sylvester Graham, and other health reformers of the time, led the way with the belief that a vegetarian diet was the best way to keep families and society "pure" and keep children from masturbating, thus saving them from sin, blindness, and an early death:

---

[*] Kellogg not only encouraged a vegetarian diet to stop sexual thoughts but also held patents on genital cages to stop children from touching themselves, circumcised boys without anesthetic, and was known to pour carbolic acid onto the clitoris of young girls found masturbating. As an extreme precaution he removed the clitoris and labia minora of anyone found to be suffering from "nymphomania."

The truth of the matter is simply this—a pure and well regulated vegetable diet, serves to take away or prevent all morbid or preternatural sexual lust, and to bring and keep the instinct more in a truly natural state, and in strict accordance with the final cause of man's sexual organization and thus enable him to be chaste in body and spirit.[6]

Certainly, before we really understood the germ theory, and made inroads into safe transportation of meat into the crowding cities using refrigeration and sterile canning techniques, there is no doubt some people did get very sick from eating meat. Eliminating unhygienic meat from the diet could legitimately have improved the health of many. But was meat the issue or did the problem have more to do with how it was stored and transported and what the meat was served with? Unfortunately, the stigma that meat is gluttonous, dirty, sinful, too "manly," leads to "animalistic" behavior, and causes disease is still present today in secular society.

In many Eastern religions, the killing of animals for meat has long been considered immoral, though many Buddhists, including the Dalai Lama himself, eat meat. While they may avoid meat, there is no Eastern religion that bans *all* animal products. Even the Jains are encouraged to be vegetarian (*not* vegan) for their health. In the West, avoiding meat was generally considered a health movement and not an ethical consideration until the 1900s.

In America there are still SDA influences behind our meat-phobic guidelines. Many of the leading authors of the 1988 official position paper on vegetarian diets published by the Association of Nutrition and Dietetics are SDA members, yet this conflict of interest was not acknowledged by the group.

When Diana was a dietetics student, she was repeatedly told that eating a Paleo-type diet was unhealthy because it "cut out food groups," yet being a vegetarian or vegan was perfectly acceptable and highly encouraged. The problem is, this idea was not based on evidence, and seems highly biased against meat because it's "bad" to eat it. This is actually where the title of the book, *Sacred Cow,* comes from. It's all too common just to assume without question that red meat is bad. But as we illustrated in the nutrition section, when you analyze the nutrient value of red meat, it's clearly one of the best sources of protein plus vitamins and minerals that are hard to find in other places.

Another group with an ideological bias against meat that is having a big impact on how the public gets nutrition information is the American College of Lifestyle Medicine, which was founded in 2004 by SDA member Dr. John Kelly. From late 2016 until October 2018 the organization's president was Dr. George Guthrie, also an SDA member. "For the treatment, reversal and prevention of lifestyle-related chronic disease, the ACLM recommends an eating plan based predominantly on a variety of minimally processed vegetables, fruits, whole grains, legumes, nuts and seeds," an ACLM press release from 2018 reads.[7] Guthrie believes that animal proteins are the primary cause of heart disease.[8]

The ACLM currently partners with several schools, including Florida State University College of Medicine, Loma Linda University, and the University of Texas, to provide the "Lifestyle Medicine Residency Curriculum" and offers online continuing medical education courses for medical professionals, plus a free syllabus to medical schools in Lifestyle Medicine. All the nutrition recommendations avoid animal proteins. You can also find speakers that will promote "sustainable health, sustainable healthcare" who claim that "Lifestyle Medicine can prevent as much as 80 percent of all chronic disease." Medical professionals attending the Lifestyle Medicine conferences can learn about how to reverse disease with low-fat, plant-based diets from leading vegan authors, sponsored by vegan processed-food companies and, of course, Loma Linda University.

There are naturally other conflicts of interest between ideology and health policy; for example, take a look at the so-called Physicians Committee for Responsible Medicine (PCRM). Although the group's name implies that it's primarily a group for doctors, fewer than 7 percent of their members have medical degrees. Led by psychiatrist and vegan activist Dr. Neal Barnard, the group offers antimeat propaganda like the benign-sounding *Good Medicine* magazine and continuing medical education courses to nurses and doctors to hand to their patients discussing how unhealthy all animal products are. PCRM advises no animal products whatsoever for babies, children, and teens.

Nurses and doctors can also download their Hospital Toolkit. The cover of this document says, "Make your hospital a leader with the American Medical Association's new 'Healthy Food Options in Hospitals' policy." This wording clearly gives the impression that the AMA endorses the PRCM policies, when this is anything but true. Actually, in a 1991 news release the AMA said that PCRM's dietary advice "could be dangerous to health and the well-being of Americans."[9] PCRM also offers a free book titled *Nutrition Guide for Clinicians* to medical students and ships cases of the book to schools. A quick flip through this book reveals how nearly every disease is caused by meat, and can be cured by a vegan diet. Former AMA president Dr. Roy Schwartz has described members of the PCRM as "neither physicians nor responsible."

The largest donor to PCRM is PETA (People for the Ethical Treatment of Animals), and both organizations support the Animal Liberation Front, which has been called one of "today's most serious domestic terrorism threats" by John E. Lewis, a deputy assistant director at the FBI. Contrary to public perception, the nonprofit organization Center for Consumer Freedom has published documents indicating that "PETA employees have killed more than 33,000 dogs, cats, puppies, and kittens since 1998."[10]

Although "no potential conflict of interest was reported by the authors," all three experts responsible for writing the official "Position of the Academy of Nutrition and Dietetics: Vegetarian Diets," Vasanto Melina, Winston Craig, and Susan Levin, are either ideological vegetarians or vegans or have a vested financial interest in an official acceptance of this diet.[11]

Vasanto Melina is described as "a consultant for individuals who would like to fine tune their plant-based diets" and is author of twelve books on vegan and vegetarian diets (including one on how to raise children on a vegetarian diet and how to eat a raw vegan diet) and is a member of the International Vegetarian Union. She also teaches plant-based cooking classes.

Winston Craig is a professor of nutrition at Andrews University, a Seventh-Day Adventist institution with the mission "to prepare dietetic and nutrition professionals for service in church, society, and the world and to influence the community at large to affirm the Seventh-day Adventist lifestyle, including the vegetarian diet." Craig is also author of several vegetarian books and research papers.

Susan Levin is the director of nutrition education for the Physicians Committee for Responsible Medicine. This is a vegan activist group described more on page 210. She has written about the importance of feeding children a vegan diet and the dangers of eating eggs. She also profits from courses for registered dietitians to earn CEUs (continuing education units) with titles like "Eating Vegan Through the Life Stages" (including how to feed children a vegan diet), "The Vegan Advantage for Athletes," and "Meat as a Risk Factor for Type 2 Diabetes."

PERSECUTION THROUGH MEAT

When governments get involved in requiring or banning certain foods, bad things can happen. Over the last few years in India, stricter laws allowing punishment for transporting or trading beef have been enacted. People are being lynched and beaten on suspicion of serving beef. The Hindu belief holds that sacred cows should never be killed, but the overall sentiment of the current right-wing Indian government is that vegetarians are good, and eating cows is evil.

Contrary to what many assume, about 75 percent of Indians eat meat, and in some states it's close to 95 percent. Although the state religion is not officially Hinduism, many would like to see it become that. A ban on beef is really a ban on Muslims; scapegoating the cow is just sleight of hand for attacking Muslims.

What's happening today in India is reminiscent of how Nazis used meat to demonize Jews.[12] As Jews economically thrived after World War I in Germany, Nazi propaganda began to focus its jealousy of their success on kosher slaughter, distorting it as an uncivilized process. Many Nazis, including Hitler, were vegetarian (or at least presented themselves as such) and saw eliminating meat from their diets as a form of purity. Jews, on the other hand, ate meat, and this was painted as "impure." Some scholars believe that this tactic elevated the Nazi party from a political one to a spiritual (and more powerful, unquestionable) one.[13]

Are we saying that those who avoid meat are equivalent to Nazis? Of course not. But what's happening in India and what happened in Germany need to be part of the ethics section of the book because today, unfortunately, this mimics the progression of the vegan movement as a progressive entity, no longer allowing us to be "primitive" and preparing us for a world without barbarity through the promise of vegetarian protein burgers produced in factories. Antimeat propaganda depicts those who eat meat as barbaric, and uncaring about animals, other humans, or the environment while avoiding meat is seen as "clean" and "pure," and these ideological biases against meat, void of concrete scientific evidence or logic, are shaping public policy. Inaccurate statistics are being repeated over and over through highly influential clickbait articles, and Facebook itself is investing in plant-based companies. There are few pushing back against these messages, and those who do are frequently harassed. Because of our position that meat is healthy, can be good for the environment, and that ethically, a diet eliminating animals could cause more harm than one that includes them, we are attacked by those who say eating and producing meat is morally aberrant, terrible for human health, and is poised to destroy the planet.

WHY CAN'T WE FIND COMMON GROUND?

If we've learned anything from the political cycle of 2016, it's that we Americans have become increasingly polarized in our worldviews. Responses ranged from opting out of friendships on social media to physical violence and death threats. We've seen the same energy in the vegan community toward ex-vegans and those who support humane animal husbandry and slaughter.

Although the goal of veganism should be less violence, we've unfortunately seen some horrific behavior from this movement. When people leave fanatical religions, the backlash is usually not pretty. Similarly, many ex-vegans have stories about losing their friends and being harassed for returning to a diet that includes meat.

Vegan bloggers who return to eating meat, usually because of failing health, often face intense opprobrium from the online vegan movement. Jordan Younger of the blog *The Blonde Vegan* received death threats when she announced that she realized her veganism was partly due to an eating disorder and that she would be incorporating dairy back into her diet again.[14] Yovanna Mendoza is another ex-vegan social media influencer who had low iron stores, lost her period, and had severe digestive issues, but when she reincorporated fish and eggs in an effort to recover her health, her community responded with hatred. Tearful "coming-out" videos are common among one-time vegan vloggers, who are only trying to save themselves from a diet that destroyed them.[15] Unfortunately, instead of having compassion for others, realizing that not all people can thrive without animal products, and allowing folks to take care of themselves, many in the vegan community dismiss them by claiming they weren't doing vegan "hard enough" and that anyone who eats meat deserves to be labeled a murderer. As members of the Paleo community, both authors can say they've never seen this sort of behavior when a Paleo blogger went keto, for example, or decided to cut out eggs, or eat some ice cream.

Perhaps even more disturbing are when vegan activists trespass and vandalize the homes and businesses of farmers and butchers.

All across America, the UK, and Australia, there have been reports of death threats, property destruction, and worse.[16] When Meredith Leigh, a young mother and expert butcher, was advertised by a primitive skills school to lead a class on humane slaughter, she received death threats against her newborn.[17] This (understandably) led her to withdraw from teaching the class—which ended up going ahead anyway, with record attendance. Another unintended boost for sales came for the owners of The Local Butcher in Berkeley, California. The owners source all their meat from farms they've personally visited in order to ensure top animal welfare standards, and list the farmers on their website. Vegan protesters from the group Direct Action Everywhere picketed for weeks, covering themselves in fake blood and wrapping themselves in plastic to look like meat, before the owners eventually relented and met the demands of the group. Their options were to either become a "vegan butchery" (when there already was one in the city), stop teaching classes (which they opposed because education is central to their mission), or to place a sign in their front window in perpetuity. They chose the sign, which says, "Attention: Animals' lives are their right. Killing them is violent and unjust, no matter how it's done." This drew international press, and the shop had their best sales month ever.[18] Meanwhile in France, butchers are now asking for protection against vegan extremists, who are vandalizing butcher shops. "If they don't want to eat meat that's their right," says Didier Tass in an NPR interview, "but imposing their beliefs on others is like a dictatorship. Imagine you work 20 years building your business and then somebody comes along and damages your shop?"[19]

In our increasingly disconnected and polarized society, love for neighbor has gone out the window in the fierce battle between "us" and the enemy "them." These religiously moral vegan extremists seem incapable of finding an ally in the fight against the industrialized food system. The antimeat ideology is strong and can often become someone's entire worldview rather than simply a dietary preference.

Unfortunately, this means that when many vegans see their health fail, they often refuse to believe it's caused by diet. As we reviewed in the nutrition section, there are seriously harmful consequences that can result from avoiding meat, even though some are able to handle this diet better than others. Again, while we respect that it's a personal choice, the morally superior posture some meat-free dieters espouse actually represents a naive view of how food is produced and, for that matter, how nature works. Life doesn't happen without death, regardless of whether you wanted it to happen.

Anyone with a modicum of awareness recognizes the horrors of factory farming. Better meat should be the goal for all of us, especially given the ecological and health arguments for well-managed animals. And because a truly sustainable food system requires animal inputs, it's not helpful to attack those of us who are fighting for better meat. The enemy is industrial agriculture and hyperpalatable infinite-shelf-life junk food, not the family of farmers down the street who wants to raise their animals on grass. Let's unify the real food community.

CHAPTER 15

WHY EAT ANIMALS IF WE COULD SURVIVE ON ONLY PLANTS?

A casual stroll through the aisles of a natural food store will reveal a smorgasbord of protein powders, plant-based burgers, and other vegan products—"food you can feel good about." They are marketed as healthier, more sustainable, and morally superior alternatives to meat.

While we understand that it can *feel* wrong to kill an animal for food, we hope we've illustrated that the emotional argument is simply illogical when considering the environmental and nutritional implications of eliminating animals from our food system. As we showed in the last chapters, creating a hierarchy of which foods are good or bad to eat is remarkably egocentric.

We also think it's highly unethical to tell someone else that they're being immoral when they consume nutrient-dense traditional food just because you don't like the idea of eating it yourself. Although well intentioned, this position may be a form of subtle classism.

While it's true that a generally plant-based diet *can* provide humans with all the nutrition they need, a diet that requires supplements poses many problems, especially for children and the poor. Will the marginalized poor of developing countries be airlifted B12, zinc, and iron supplements? How about rural communities and lower-income families?

IS "LESS MEAT" A FEASIBLE OPTION FOR EVERYONE? IS AVOIDING MEAT A PRIVILEGED OPTION?

By opting out of the meat system, are people really going to change how animals are produced? Are "Eat Less Meat" and "Meatless Mondays" campaigns helping our health and the environment? They're certainly effective at perpetuating the myth that all meat is unsustainable and unhealthy, but are they changing our production methods? Or perhaps these campaigns are actually obscuring the discussion.

In fact, as we have seen, there are major vitamin deficiencies connected to a meatless diet. With 1.62 billion people worldwide suffering from anemia, and red meat as our best source of bioavailable iron, we need to take an honest look at how we vilify meat for health reasons.

The Meatless Mondays campaign that recently took over the NYC public schools raises serious concerns. First, the campaigners are using meat as a nutritional scapegoat. By eliminating all meat on Mondays, the campaign is encouraging over 1.1 million students in the largest school district in the country to believe nutrient-dense animal-based foods are unhealthy and bad for the environment. The vast majority of these kids are food insecure, with 10 percent of them homeless and approximately 75 percent qualifying for free or reduced-price school lunch. A powerful and often overlooked aspect of both early and later life achievement is adequate nutrition in childhood—meat and animal products could arguably take center stage. In chapter six we discussed the only study looking at supplementing at-risk kids with more meat, and the ones who got the meat supplement scored higher academically, behaviorally, and physically. And as we referenced on page 98, eliminating all meat from the US food system would only eliminate GHG emissions by 2.6 percent, while increasing nutrient deficiencies. Given that background, does it make sense to reduce meat for these kids?

Is the problem in the public schools the burgers, or could it actually be (ironically "plant-based") fries, pizza, tater tots, chips, and cookies? Is it OK for these programs to post their antimeat misinformation in schools, telling many food-insecure kids that giving up meat is the right thing to do?

It's important to step back for a minute and realize that those who have the choice to avoid a nutrient-dense food are only able to do so in a well-fed state. Avoiding meat is a privilege that many people simply don't have. Most of the world's population is not able to push away a nutritious food option. In many places, adequate nutrition can't be obtained from plants alone because only animals can thrive in the local environment. If you remember from the environmental section, high-quality cropland with adequate water to produce vegetables isn't available everywhere.

LIVESTOCK ARE CRITICAL TO MANY IN DEVELOPING COUNTRIES

In her book *Defending Beef*, Nicolette Hahn Niman also points out the important concept that domestic animals are of huge importance in terms of nutrition and food security in developing countries. Many people living in poverty depend on livestock, and eliminating animals from the food system would actually increase hunger and poverty, leading to more people relying on the government for food assistance. "In contrast with crop farming, which produces sporadic, seasonal, perishable products, livestock is an asset that can be maintained for short or long periods of time then quickly converted to food or cash when needed." Since crop farming requires not only good land but harvest at a specific time, it's a far less reliable and insecure source of food. Animals are also mobile—think about how important that is to someone who doesn't have the money to own land. They also require less attention and resources than cropping and can multiply on their own (no need to buy seeds from Monsanto!). Nutritionally, these people also benefit dramatically from including animal products in their diet.

More than 820 million people are suffering from hunger, and nutrient deficiencies are a serious concern throughout the world. About half the 767 million people living in extreme poverty depend on raising animals for food or for their income. Is it ethical, then, to tell a hungry or poor person who raises meat that they should avoid meat because a well-fed Westerner doesn't feel it's OK? Could claiming moral superiority over those who do eat meat be itself an act of extreme privilege and an insult to all people from cultures that have traditionally eaten animal products?

When we advocate that folks give up meat wholesale, we're often not recommending they fill that hole in their diets with nutritious food. What's the most affordable food source? As we've seen, it's those processed carbohydrate foods. Instead of worrying about how much meat everyone will be eating, we should be *very* worried about how much junk food they're eating. A diet high in refined grains (e.g., processed foods) is the biggest nutritional contributor to diabetes in China.[1] Fast-food chains in China have a growth rate of 11.1 percent annually, a $175 billion market in 2018.[2] Yum China Holdings, which owns KFC, Pizza Hut, and Taco Bell, plans to add fifteen thousand more restaurants in China over the next fifteen years. According to the Food and Agriculture Organization, rice, corn, and wheat make up more than 50 percent of our food, and 75 percent of our diet comes from only twelve crops.[3]

An interesting case study of what happens when meat and fat are replaced with processed foods is that of the native Arctic population called the Yamalo-Nenets. Owing to several changes in their environment and lifestyle, their diets have shifted drastically to include cheap, highly processed carbohydrates like packaged noodles, whereas before they ate few carbohydrates and relied on fat and meat as their primary calorie source. With this change, there have been staggering increases in obesity and chronic diseases never before seen in this population that traditionally ate mostly venison and fish.[4]

In northern Quebec, government officials said they worked closely with the Nunavik to develop a culturally appropriate food guide. One look at the "food igloo" inside the Nunavik Food Guide (written by Canadian dietitians) says so much about how wrong we are. It would be hard to illustrate a more perfect metaphor for the entire nutrition debacle. They're advised to eat seven to ten servings from the "vegetables, berries, and fruit" group, and this includes orange juice, bananas, watermelon, and grapes. In the guide, Raisin Bran is on the list of recommended grain products to be consumed six to eight times a day. Way up at the top of the food igloo, in the smallest category, are the foods most traditional to their culture—and the guide recommends these be eaten just two to three times a day.[5]

The *Nunavik Inuit Health Survey 2004* shows that approximately 60 percent of the adult population is overweight or obese, which was a sharp increase over the previous survey conducted in 1992. Their intake of traditional foods, obtained by fishing and hunting, declined to only 16 percent of energy intake in 2004, compared to 21 percent in 1992. Iron deficiency anemia affects over half the nonpregnant women in Nunavik. The iron status of women of childbearing age and pregnant women is also considered at a critical level, and this can lead to significant developmental issues with babies. Interestingly, in the guidelines they're told in one sentence to purchase lean meats like chicken and turkey but then are also told that seal meat (which is definitely not low in fat) is one of the best sources of iron.

One study of 245 children in ten communities of Nunavik showed that although traditional foods contributed a very low percentage of their total intake (only 2.6 percent), those who consumed these foods, which were mainly caribou and Arctic char, were significantly more nourished, and at the same time, they consumed fewer total calories and carbohydrates.[6] These foods contributed protein, omega-3 fatty acids, iron, phosphorus, zinc, copper, selenium, niacin, pantothenic acid, riboflavin, and vitamin B12. Why then are we recommending orange juice and other tropical foods, which are high in sugar and relatively low in nutrients, and putting their traditional foods in the red category when these foods are among the most nutrient-dense and lowest-calorie foods available to humans? Is this ethical? Sustainable?

EVERYTHING EATS AND IS EATEN

To want to end factory farming is a fantastic goal that we fully support. To want "least harm" is also important. The problem is, when we refuse to accept how nature works, and try to eliminate animals from our food system, our food system will collapse. A truly resilient food system requires as much life as possible, and this means animals *and* plants. Life feeds on death. To remove ourselves from death is to remove ourselves from the cycle of life. We cannot bypass the laws of nature. We're dependent on all living things, yet we like to think we can somehow survive with less life surrounding us.

Many people have personal reasons against eating meat. However, the environmental, nutrition, sentience, and least-harm arguments appear tenuous at best. Lab meat, fake meat, and other "clean" proteins are not, in fact, better options. Instead, photosynthesis, respecting natural cycles, and increasing biodiversity should be the answer.

If you imagine the planet without humans, there would actually be much *more* life. If we destroy ourselves, life on this planet would go on. Animals will continue to eat plants and other animals; the rhythm of nature will carry on. Our decisions right now about what kind of impact we want to have on the planet will simply determine whether humans will be part of Earth's future.

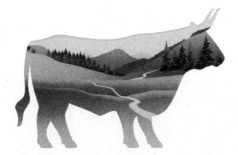

PART IV

WHAT WE CAN DO

CHAPTER 16

FEEDING THE WORLD

We believe we have made a sound case that it is difficult to produce optimum human health with a plant-only diet, particularly in the very young, very old, and at-risk populations such as the poor and marginalized minorities. For well-to-do twenty- to thirty-somethings, who have the privilege of pushing away a nutrient-dense food like red meat, a plant-only diet may work during the prime of life. It may offer health benefits relative to hyperpalatable, industrial foods, but it is not the only option and is unlikely to be the best option.

We have also made the case that a food system absent animal inputs is unsustainable because it relies upon synthetic fertilizers (and a host of related agrichemicals) that are collectively destroying our topsoil. On the ethics front we have explored the principle of least harm and the fact that all life feeds on life. A vegan diet is not a bloodless diet, and may even destroy more life than a regenerative, pasture-centric model. Although each of these topics must first be considered in isolation, they must eventually be stitched together and considered as a whole.

Perhaps the ultimate manifestation of that holistic analysis is the topic of feeding the world.

If our food system (1) makes people so sick that their health-care costs bankrupt global economies, and (2) destroys our topsoil such that we can effectively no longer produce food, then it is, by definition, unsustainable. We firmly believe that a sustainable food system is one that can both feed the populace well and stand the test of time.

We know your burning question: *This all sounds great, Diana and Robb, but can we feed the world this way?* Please bear with us for a few more pages because this is a complex and loaded question. Let's consider a few more questions before we delve into how to feed the world . . .

WHAT IS EFFICIENT FOOD PRODUCTION?

Many processes are assessed on "efficiency," as if that process occurs in a universe all its own. True efficiency may not be the absolute maximum yield we can get from a corn harvest but rather a maximization of a host of healthy, nutritious food products, a reduction in heat production from barren ground, and improved water and carbon retention—to name but a few considerations. We fail to see how products like lab meat or ultraprocessed plant-based meat alternatives (twice the price of grass-fed beef), reliant on chemically grown monocrops, improve ecosystem function and sequester carbon.

In addition to considering the food production potential of a given approach, we must also look at energy considerations and the often-overlooked externalities of these processes. If the discussion is lacking these nuances, the solutions proposed may appear compelling, but often miss knock-on effects and externalities.

HOW MANY PEOPLE CAN THE EARTH SUPPORT?

Some estimates suggest that the carrying capacity of the earth is as little as three million people. Carrying capacity is the theoretical number of people our planet can sustain indefinitely. This seems a stretch, though, as the global population in 10,000 BC is estimated to have been between one and fifteen million. Recent projections have put the number (somewhat inconveniently) at seven billion. The reality is, no one really knows what this number is and both the optimists and pessimists in the world could probably benefit from a dose of honesty.

Ironically, the most concerning factor in the climate change story—fossil fuels—have remained a problem mainly because their prices have plummeted over time. Multiple predictions of peak oil have been made, only to recede into the past without being realized. This is a nontrivial point: since the 1960s certain camps have been warning that we are destined to imminently run out of oil, and when that happens the global economy will collapse. Only . . . the day that we're supposed to run out of oil never seems to arrive. While oil is a finite resource, every scientific prediction thus far has proved wrong. Quietly, the narrative has shifted; now, some have suggested that we have too much oil.[1]

The point to all this is that the doomsday prophets have not produced a good showing. The authors find themselves in the uncomfortable position of generally being in the "optimist" camp, acknowledging that freedom, innovation, and trade have done more to improve the lot of humanity than any well-meaning oligarchy or dictator ever did. That said, we do see some areas of challenge when we overlay a food system that makes our populace sick while destroying our topsoil.

The antimeat camps raise concern about how much food is diverted away from people toward the "inefficient" process of feeding animals. (As we showed in previous chapters, this is not only a misrepresentation but largely a false pretense. If folks were truly concerned about this topic, they would picket ethanol and alcohol producers, not ranchers.) The concern about how we'll feed the world is well placed, but again, within the antimeat camps it is not hard to find vocal proponents of draconian population control. Apparently, there are too many people in the world and the "science is settled." But which is the real problem, too many people or too little food? What's more, seemingly no one from these camps ever talks about what *does* reduce birthrates: sound property rights, a (reasonably) transparent legal system, and an educated populace, specifically women.[2] This process is well studied and well validated yet appears nowhere in the talking points of the antimeat crowd. Why?

All of that is a bit of a long-winded way of saying: no one really knows what the carrying capacity of the earth is. It's certainly something to consider, but it's likely not prudent to perform a massive sociopolitical engineering project on a process that is infinitely complex.

SHOULD WE PRODUCE "FEED" OR NUTRIENT-DENSE FOOD?

A paper published in *Nature* in December 2018 looked at current worldwide nutrient deficiencies by country. The researchers found that we're doing great at carbohydrate production, but not as well with protein and other micronutrients.[3] We need to stop thinking about producing enough calories and start to consider how to produce enough nutrients. The authors found that we will continue to be able to produce enough human "feed" until 2050, but in an opinion letter in the *Washington Post*, coauthor Gerald C. Nelson, a professor emeritus at the University of Illinois at Urbana-Champaign and a former senior research fellow at the International Food Policy Research Institute, said the following:

> *Our success with carbohydrates, however, has had a serious downside: a worldwide plague of obesity, diabetes and other diet-related diseases. The World Health Organization reports that in 2014, there were 462 million underweight adults worldwide but more than 600 million who were obese—nearly two-thirds*

*of them in developing countries. And childhood obesity is rising
much faster in poorer countries than in richer ones. Meanwhile,
micronutrient shortages such as Vitamin A deficiency are already
causing blindness in somewhere between 250,000 and 500,000
children a year and killing half of them within 12 months of them
losing their sight. Dietary shortages of iron, zinc, iodine and folate
all have devastating health effects. These statistics point to the
need for more emphasis on nutrients other than carbohydrates in
our diets.[4]*

To shift our discussion on food security from "calories" to
"nutrient security" means we have to seriously question how we
are to provide some of the most critical nutrients. We're simply not
going to solve our diabetes and obesity epidemics with more rice,
corn, and wheat. The food system we advocate for, one with more
well-managed grazing animals, is both more nutrient dense and better for the environment.

WHAT IS THE ENVIRONMENTAL FOOTPRINT OF A DIET OF "FEED"?

Using a life cycle analysis approach, one recent study looking at
sixty thousand households in Japan found that meat consumption
was not the main indicator of high food-related carbon footprints.[5]
The households with the highest carbon footprints were ones that
consumed more fish, vegetables, alcohol, and sugary foods, and ate
out at restaurants most often. Meat consumption was a much lower
contributor compared to the most glaring offender: eating out.

When we vilify red meat, a nutrient-dense real food, does this
mean we get a free pass for nutrient-poor, ultraprocessed foods that
we know are driving disease? What are the other emissions consequences resulting from a poor diet? What are the health-care emissions of diabetes, for example?

Just in America, the necessary one to four insulin injections
per day for treating diabetics results in thirteen million needles and

syringes per day. There are also lancets, insulin pump tubing, continuous glucose monitoring tubing, and insertion devices to take into account. Much of the time, these items are flushed down the toilet. Although there's no national program for safe needle disposal, patients can send their medical waste to a materials recovery facility to be sorted. What can't be recycled is brought to a landfill. During the expensive process of sorting, sanitation workers are at high risk for needle-stick injuries (there's currently no system to track the number of injuries, or related infections this can cause).[6]

One of the medical conditions that can result from diabetes is kidney failure. Hemodialysis is the process of artificially replacing kidney function in order to filter blood once the kidneys can no longer perform this function, and it requires large amounts of water, medical supplies, and energy. In the US, 450,000 people need dialysis. A typical patient undergoing dialysis uses about eighteen thousand liters of water and 800 to 925 kilowatt-hours of energy per year, and produces over seven billion pounds of medical waste.[7]

Though there are few cradle-to-grave papers looking into the total environmental impact of the results of a bad diet, you can probably imagine the tremendous resources a disease like type 2 diabetes can cost. There's also the large amounts of gauze and other materials needed to treat the amputations and gaping wounds caused by diabetes, and the transportation required for frequent hospital visits. All these services require staff, energy, antibiotics, large amounts of plastic, and time off by family caregivers. Much of this could be avoided if we had a healthier population that ate well. So while hospitals are now touting their reduction in meat as an environmentally positive step, given the fact that most patients in hospitals require more nutrient density and protein to recover, perhaps the focus should instead be on helping people improve their poor diets and lifestyles and avoid hospitals in the first place. But, cynically, where's the profit in that? The reality is, reducing meat in hospitals saves tons of money, and we suspect that hospitals are prioritizing their bottom line over the general health of our population.

The narrative put forward by meat-phobic nutrition advocates places the blame for all this cost and misery almost exclusively on animal products. These are items that folks are eating less of, not more. And let's not forget that in controlled trials (DIETFITS, A TO Z, and others), meat-inclusive diets, be they low fat or low carb, showed a reversal of insulin resistance and type 2 diabetes so long as folks reduced their consumption of refined foods.

ARE LAB MEAT AND MEAT ALTERNATIVES VIABLE SOLUTIONS?

Lab meat is more about intellectual property and profits than about health, ethics, or the environment. It's convenient for them that many in the plant-based movement are behind them, as it provides the illusion that these foods are "clean"—whatever they are, they're anything but "real." Meat alternatives are ways of further processing raw ingredients and making larger profits from highly destructive agricultural practices. We should also be questioning the ethics of people pushing a system that requires so many chemical inputs, ruins soil health, and expands the gap between people and their food producers.

At the end of the day, we just don't see meat produced in bioreactors as a win for anyone other than the people making the lab meat. Farmers are still getting paid low rates for their commodities while destroying the soil, more energy is needed to turn soy and corn into meat than what can be done in nature with an animal, and we're doing this all in the name of "least harm"? Remember Grassworld from chapter seven? Lab meat is the opposite of the direction we need to be moving in.

Luckily, we know of self-replicating natural bioreactors that upcycle food we can't eat on land we can't crop into nutrient-dense protein while increasing biodiversity, improving the water-holding capacity of the soil, and sequestering carbon . . .

DO WE HAVE THE LAND FOR ALL-GRASS-FED BEEF?

Now that we've outlined how our current system and many of the proposed solutions are neither healthier nor better for the planet, the big question can be addressed: Do we have the land for it? Diana consulted with a few experts to run the numbers, including Dr. Allen Williams, an ecosystem and soil health consultant, farmer, and former agriculture professor who is an advocate for regenerative agriculture. She also spoke with Dr. Jason Rowntree from Michigan State, Jim Howell of Grasslands, LLC, and Dr. John Ikerd, a prolific writer, agricultural economist, and retired professor emeritus from the University of Missouri.

One critical piece of information to keep in mind is to remember that we're comparing industrial monocropping to regenerative agriculture, which have drastically different impacts on the land. Even though it takes more land to produce well-managed grass-finished beef, it could be argued that the regenerative solution is a smarter one for our future than the chemical one. At a recent conference about grass-fed beef, Rowntree said in his presentation, **"I'd rather have 2.5 acres of regenerative agriculture than 1 acre of extractive agriculture."**

Let that sink in for a moment.

OK, let's dive into what sort of acres we'd need in the US to finish all our beef herd on grass. In the thought experiment we are about to embark on, the numbers are rough and could certainly be challenged, but it's a good place to start a discussion. If you remember from page 150, when looking at the life cycle of beef cattle, these animals all start out grazing and are either finished at a feedlot or finished on grass. If we look at the current amount of idle grassland, underutilized pasture, and cropland that would be freed up from grain production in an all-grass-finished scenario, the short answer to our question is yes. We do have the land to finish all our current beef cattle on pasture in the US. Here's how:

To finish moderate-frame cattle, bringing them from 800 to 1,200 pounds, it takes on average approximately one acre per animal on productive pasture, assuming a weight gain of two pounds per day over six to seven months. Managers shoot for around a twenty-five-pound intake of pasture a day for each steer. In the US there are approximately twenty-nine million cattle currently being finished in a feedlot per year (this includes domestic and export markets).[8]

If we are now grass-finishing all beef cattle produced annually in the US, we can reduce the ninety to ninety-four million acres of corn planted. Approximately 36–40 percent of today's corn crop actually goes into livestock feed (cattle, pigs, and chickens), with the rest being used mainly for high-fructose corn syrup and ethanol. While cattle consume dried distiller's grains, a by-product of alcohol production, that by-product is included in the percentage allocated to "livestock." The point being, converting the crop acres back into grass is not any threat to food security. As we mentioned in chapter ten, only 10–13 percent of a typical beef steer's diet is actually grain.

OK, back to our numbers. If we take just fifteen million acres of cornfields and consider these productive (after all, they once were thriving grasslands), each of them can finish 1.25 steers per acre. Altogether, these acres finish 18.75 million cattle.

In addition to converting some of our corn acres back to grassland, there are over five hundred million acres of privately owned pastureland in the US,[9] and many experts we've spoken to estimate it's only being utilized at 30 percent capacity. This leaves enormous potential for better grazing management. If we were able to use just 10 percent (fifty million acres) and conservatively assume it would only produce 10 million cattle, we're now up to 28.75 million cattle that we can finish on grass.

Interestingly, there are also other opportunities for land. If we could graze just 30 percent of the current twenty million acres of land locked up in the Conservation Reserve Program, a program that pays farmers to allow the land to grow fallow, this land that is currently not allowed to be grazed except in an emergency could give us an additional six million acres. Though it would not be as productive as the former cropland, it could still yield approximately four million beef cattle, increasing our number to 32.75 million cattle finished on grass, which is more than the current beef herd finished in feedlots.*

But because grass-finished cattle are not fed a high-energy diet (compared to the feedlot), their carcasses are generally 20–30 percent lighter. While a large component of this is excessive fat trim, the differences in productivity should be accounted for. Therefore, hypothetically, 30 percent more cows would be needed.

However, experts in regenerative grazing practices like Jim Howell report an increase in stocking rates (the number of animals the land can support) by 50–100 percent. If we go with a conservative 30 percent assumed increase in productivity from typical grazing to better management, this accounts for the increase in cowherd size. Similar data from Michigan State University reported a 30 percent increase in overall productivity of converting to regenerative grazing practices as well.

Not only could it be possible to finish all US beef cattle on grass, but grass-finishing beef is more profitable as well. Today's corn farmer grosses about $680 per acre while in a wholesale market one grass-finished steer goes for $1,600. There are also fewer inputs (no chemical fertilizers, herbicides, seeds, or heavy equipment). You do need more labor to move them (which creates more jobs), but overall, the net profit to the rancher is higher with well-managed cattle (and less money to corporate chemical agriculture giants). And again, these acres will be a net gain to our agricultural land because they would be beneficial to our ecosystems instead of destroying them. Current government regulations of industrial animal feeding operations fail to protect the natural environment or public health, and government-guaranteed loans and tax breaks incentivize new and expanding CAFO operations. Fundamental shifts in government programs could easily shift the profit potential of beef production

---

* A side benefit of allowing this land to be regeneratively grazed would be the increase in wildlife habitat, soil health, and overall ecosystem function. Why not have a "permanent land-use easement" on all land going into the CRP program that allows for regenerative grazing and prohibits plowing and crop production?

to ranchers and grazers who produce grass-based beef, providing opportunities for more independent beef producers.

More grass-finished beef not only means healthier land but also healthier local economies. Profits made from the current CAFO meat industry mostly go to corporate integrators, rather than the ranchers who raise the cattle. These profits are primarily the result of government programs that ensure a dependable supply of feed grains that are often supplied at prices less than farmers' cost to produce them. Across the US, the small towns that once supported the farms were vibrant because of farming and ranching. Today, there are fewer family farms left, and more towns are boarded-up shells of what they used to be. It seems that unless there's a university or tourist attraction, the local businesses are struggling. If we continue down the road of even more industrial-scale agriculture, this will only get worse. Farmers need to make a profit, but under our current system many farmers planting out their corn crop know they'll be underwater by harvest time. But their hands are tied. It doesn't have to be like this. More regenerative agriculture means healthier people, communities, economies, soil, water cycles, and mineral cycles, and more wildlife.

Does this mean the entire world will or needs to shift to grass-fed beef as the primary protein source? That's not what we're saying. Different regions have area-specific ecosystems that can provide different foods. In some areas it may make more sense to raise camels or goats, depending on what the landscape can provide. When we see regions feeding themselves instead of relying on outside food, we generally see more resilience. Animals play an important role in all regenerative food systems, as well as healthy diets for humans. The goal should be to help local farmers and ranchers learn to care for their land in a way that will result in healthy food and best agricultural practices. We can produce more nutrient-dense food in this way. Our current reliance on industrially produced chemical grain production to "feed the world" is the opposite of this. Malnutrition in "less-developed" areas of the world is a reflection of ecologically degraded agricultural systems as well as dysfunctional governments.

Hunger is largely a political issue, not a food production issue. When people have better access to land, loans, and markets, we all win. The organization Heifer International is a great example of what could be done to address global hunger.

WHAT CHANGES WOULD BE NEEDED TO MAKE A MORE REGENERATIVE FOOD SYSTEM HAPPEN?

How can this shift take place? It would require some big changes to policies on several levels. But, being optimists, we want to believe it's possible. The first major shift needs to be from reductionism to a more holistic approach. Even looking at "reduction in emissions" as a goal is, as we've illustrated, missing the nutritional and over-all ecosystem benefits we see from well-managed ruminant animals grazing on uncroppable land. Keep in mind this overemphasis on "reducing emissions" (absent context) leads to goofy ideas like we should have fewer shellfish in the oceans.

On the policy level, how about we incentivize farmers who increase ecosystem health? One of the challenges of narrowly focusing on emissions is that we're losing sight of the larger goals: more biodiversity, healthier environments, better soil that can hold water, and agriculture that is appropriate to the landscape (no flood-irrigated almonds in areas that have water shortages).

Governments need to stop incentivizing overproduction of nutrient-poor foods that destroy the environment. There are a variety of ideas being put forth on how farmers could actually benefit from better environmental practices, including carbon credits for ranchers who are raising cattle in a regenerative way. One of the great aspects of raising better meat is that it's also better for a farmer's bank account. Consumers can help create more of a demand by purchasing their meat from producers who are using regenerative techniques.

As we illustrated, there does seem to be enough land in the US to grass-finish all our beef cattle. Farmers can also "stack enterprises." In this way, the land used for cattle becomes multiuse. For example, mobile chickens can follow behind the cattle, and cattle can be grazing a harvested corn field. Using land for crops and grazing and egg production is not only efficient but more profitable and actually better for soil health.

We need to stop producing human "feed" and focus on nourishing people with nutrient-dense food. On the dietary guidelines side of the equation, given the fact that we don't know what a global diet is—but we do know that nutrient-poor, ultraprocessed foods are the main issue—how about coming up with a recommendation to eat less ultraprocessed food? Brazil's guidelines are a good example of this. We can bring back cooking classes to schools and community centers, and run campaigns recommending families get back in the kitchen to eat more real food.

Instead of "everything in moderation," it's time we start recognizing that obesity in the West is the result of "quick, convenient, and cheap," which have been the driving forces in our food system. Our food policies have been determined by economic interests from the agri-food industry. The factory farming of animals is a consequence of this drive to produce more fast, cheap food and is the root cause of the current backlash against animal agriculture. Moving forward, the ecological needs of our entire food system will necessitate a return to farming in a more natural way. This will also result in more nutrient-dense foods for humans and a healthier population.

RESILIENT, REGIONAL FOOD SYSTEMS

The goal of any resilient food system should be regional reliance. Many of our foreign food aid policies actually harm local economies. Don't misunderstand, it's completely reasonable to help out those in an emergency, but most people don't understand the huge disservice we're doing to countries when we continue to send them free nutrient-poor food. There's a lot of money to be made in the industry of aid.

Michael Matheson Miller's film *Poverty, Inc.* shows many examples of this. In the film, Peter Greer, CEO of Hope International, talks about what he saw in Rwanda. A church in Atlanta decided that it was going to send over eggs to a small town in Rwanda after the genocide. This seems like a great way to help, right? But the unintended consequences were huge.

A local man had just recently started a small egg business. It was a big investment for him. Just as his business was taking off, a flood of surplus free eggs from this church in Atlanta came into town and crushed his business. The next year, when the church decided to focus its energy in other ways, there were no longer local eggs. The Atlanta church egg donations actually had a long-term negative effect on this community. All too often the desire to "do good" needs to be tempered with an understanding of unintended consequences.

A similar situation happened in Haiti, which they're now struggling to correct. After the earthquake of 2010, we began dumping our surplus rice on the Haitian people; we not only altered their diet but actually hampered their ability to feed themselves, as they largely abandoned producing their own food. Former president Bill Clinton has officially apologized for subsidy policies made during his time in office that he now sees were a huge mistake.

When countries can no longer feed themselves and have to rely on imports, it makes them extremely vulnerable. Venezuela is a good example of this. When the price of oil was high, farmers left the fields and the country gradually started importing the majority of its food. However, when the price of oil fell, everything crumbled. In a statement made on February 9, 2018, UN human rights experts warned, "Vast numbers of Venezuelans are starving, deprived of essential medicines, and trying to survive in a situation that is spiraling downwards with no end in sight."[10]

Resilient food systems on a regional level that are less reliant on fossil fuels, chemicals, and other outside imports are necessary in order for countries to be stable. The world needs regenerative agriculture now more than ever. The systems that get implemented may look different depending on the region's specific resources. This is an ironic point in the current climate of concern over cultural appropriation and respect for cultural identity. Is it our job to tell those who rely on animal products for critical nutrients that they should stop eating meat and adopt a vegan diet because we're uncomfortable with the idea of death? A far more respectful position is to encourage the concept of food sovereignty, a term coined by members of Via Campesina in 1996. It means people have the right to healthy and culturally appropriate food produced through ecologically sound and sustainable methods, and a right to define their own food and agricultural systems. Instead of top-down regulations on what food production should look like, the food sovereignty movement encourages a "bottom-up" approach, allowing for more local control over which food will suit a particular region and culture best.[11]

The solutions may entail cattle grazing on grasslands in the American West but will likely include goats, sheep, and camels in more arid regions. On Diana's farm they host interns from around the world, and many from the sacred valley in Peru, where not many vegetables grow. There aren't twenty-four-hour grocery stores or even much electricity, so a large animal that requires cold storage doesn't make tons of sense. For them, *cuyes* (guinea pigs) have been a favorite source of protein for the last five thousand years. Because they're small, they can be consumed in one meal. Like cattle, guinea pigs (although they're monogastric) are also great at "upcycling nutrients," turning hay and greens into nutrient-dense meat. So while the concept of eating guinea pigs may seem unappealing to many readers, both authors feel it is not our place to impose our food preferences on others. Sustainability and healthy, delicious food looks like many different things in different areas. It's all about context.

Will all this change tomorrow? Realistically not, sadly, especially with the current farm subsidies in place. The government is basically guaranteeing a cheap, environmentally destructive food system that is making us sick. It's laughable that a sugar tax is being considered as we are subsidizing the corn syrup industry. When a full accounting is considered, Silicon Valley's obsession with lab meats is ridiculous. But people like simple stories, and the money to be made in selling grass-fed beef produced in regional food systems is largely with the producers, not big agriculture. In today's black-and-white world, complexity and nuance have been lost.

We need to start looking at sustainability as not just ecological integrity but also societal well-being. This means finding ecologically sound ways of meeting the nutritional needs of people. Humans are an integral part of nature. We should strive to live in harmony with nature. If we succeed in doing so, we will thrive, and so will the planet. It's time to stop looking at the earth as a resource "for us" and instead see it as a habitat for all.

WHAT CAN I DO?

There are a lot of things we as individuals can do to live healthier and more sustainable lives. Many aren't food related, but because nutrition is our wheelhouse and counts for a large part of human health, we'll be spending the most time on how to improve your diet.

Our "disposable" culture is certainly not great for the environment. Better than swapping steak for salad would be buying less single-use "stuff," gadgets you likely don't really need, and cheap "fast fashion" that is worn once then tossed or donated, which actually can cause a ton of other issues.

We imported over $5 billion of vegetables (mostly in the form of tomatoes, onions, and bell peppers), $1.5 billion of avocados, and $2.9 billion of beer from Mexico in 2017. Is drinking Mexican beer with a side of guacamole "cleaner" than eating locally sourced grass-fed beef? We're not hearing much about the high carbon footprint of avocados, nor about the destructive agricultural practices needed to produce this monocrop. Who harvested those tomatoes and how were they treated? What was the total environmental cost of your salad in the winter, and was it truly more ethical or nutrient dense than a grass-fed steak?

We've come up with some easy steps you can take to improve.

KEEP YOUR DOLLARS LOCAL

Shopping locally and supporting food producers who are doing it right is not only healthier and better for the environment; it also supports local economies. When you buy things from multinational corporations, very little of your money actually supports the person who grew or made that product. If we want to maintain vibrant small towns and communities, it's critical that we circulate our money in our own regions. You'll keep families employed and also get fresher, healthier food.

AVOID DEBT

Although this is not really within the scope of our book, we both feel strongly that living within your means and not being a financial burden on society is critical to a sustainable world. Buying things we don't need (and can't afford) creates a huge carbon footprint, and debt is not only stressful—it's wasteful. Most of us in Western societies have way more junk than we need, and most of these items are not necessary or even made domestically. Keeping your purchases to a minimum, and investing in higher-quality, domestically produced goods is better for the environment and for your pocketbook. This is particularly important when it comes to clothing. One pair of jeans or a cotton T-shirt that might cost less than twenty dollars has a massive environmental impact. Buy used and prioritize higher-quality clothes made from regenerative fibers like wool.

GET INVOLVED WITH YOUR FOOD

Growing your own food or volunteering at a local farm is one of the healthiest hobbies. Victory gardens were popular during World War II when the country faced food shortages. Diana's farm has hosted gyms to do "farm fit"–type workouts and also offers "work-for-share" programs where folks can help out on the farm in exchange for vegetables. This is a win-win for everyone, and let me tell you, real farmer's carries are no joke! Check out Diana's book

The Homegrown Paleo Cookbook for a full guide to growing (and cooking) your own healthy food. Diana also describes the importance of hunters to ecological health in her book, and we highly encourage readers to consider taking a course and learning more about it.

If you're not physically able to hunt or do farm work, maybe you have another skill that would benefit the farm, like graphic design or accounting. If you're on a local planning board, try to use your influence to make agriculture more feasible in your area. Many places have strict zoning laws and other rules that make it really difficult for small-scale farms to do business. Stronger local governments that are agriculturally friendly make a huge difference. Many of the rules set by the national government intended for large commercial farms are not applicable to small-scale regenerative farms and actually hinder their success. Preventing the overdevelopment of land and conserving spaces in order to have farming is also critical to keeping regional food systems thriving.

CONTRIBUTE TO REGENERATIVE AGRICULTURE ORGANIZATIONS

Have the means to make a difference? Donate to one of our favorite nonprofits dedicated to the production and education about better meat. Visit Sacredcow.info for an up-to-date list!

SHOW YOUR KIDS HOW REAL FOOD IS GROWN

Introduce your kids to farming and food production. Kids who spend more time in nature are more likely to become conservationists in the future. On our farm we host school groups in the hopes that once these kids grow up they'll remember how much they loved their visits to the farm and will be more likely to save farmland from being developed into shopping malls and housing. One note: while urban farms are great gardens, they often do not incorporate animals into their fertility program. If you can, seek out a farm that actually raises animals and vegetables, so your kids can see how animals are a critical part of a regenerative farm, and so they don't

learn that vegetables just magically come out of the ground without animal inputs.

FOLLOW A HEALTHY LIFESTYLE

Keeping yourself healthy reduces your individual burden on society, and it happens to make for a much more pleasurable way to live. In addition to diet, there are quite a few things you can do in order to improve your health. Getting adequate sleep is probably the most important factor. Even on a perfect diet, if your sleep isn't dialed in, your brainpower will suffer and excess weight can be an issue. Movement, as I'm sure you know, is also really important to overall health, as is time in nature, having meaningful relationships with others, and having a "why." A reason to get up in the morning, for something larger than you, is an important factor in longevity. This might mean your children, a hobby, your work, or some other passion.

By far, the single greatest thing you can do for your health is to change your diet, preparing real food in your own home. In the next chapter we'll lay out what we've found to be the optimal template for a nutrient-dense yet sustainable diet for humans.

CHAPTER 17

EAT LIKE A NUTRIVORE

We know you must be wondering what we feel is the ideal diet. In this chapter we'll walk you through it, including guidelines for a thirty-day challenge to get you started.

As you might have guessed, we think there is nuance to this topic. As we have said, *there isn't just one specific macronutrient ratio, ideal food, or way of eating for all humans.* We believe, however, that many people can benefit from eating fewer calories and processed foods and incorporating healthy animal products in the form of meat, eggs, or dairy. We also feel that if you'd like a starting point, prioritizing protein while keeping micronutrients high and overall calories in check is a great way to eat. Some people who wish to lose weight may want to go lower in overall calories while keeping protein and micronutrients high. This is similar to what is known as a protein-sparing modified fast.

Many have used this type of diet successfully but have failed to consider the importance of food-based micronutrients and sustainability as part of the picture. Pulling all these facets together appears to be the golden ticket to an optimal human diet. We'll call this

combination of healthy choices and locally sourced options "eating like a nutrivore."*

Although the idea of this, similar to a Paleo diet, was to focus on the most nutrient-dense foods available to us in our modern world, the image of cavemen and a false image of a "meat-only" diet seems to have turned some people off.

We suggest a thirty-day introduction where you are eating 100 percent nutrient-dense food, with no sweeteners of any kind, then transitioning to 80-20—80 percent Paleo foods, and 20 percent healthy, non-Paleo options. We also recommend buying the best-produced food you have access to.

Both of us have recommended similar thirty-day resets and "Paleo challenges" to our clients, which have included the general population as well as Fortune 50 companies and governmental institutions. We also endorse the Whole30 program, which is similar to Paleo and can be life changing. For others, the keto diet is the ticket. What the Nutrivore Challenge and all these other plans have in common is prioritizing protein to avoid ravenous hunger and reducing your intake of highly processed foods, which are easy to overeat. Some folks jump in with both feet, others start by "just" eliminating sugary beverages (this can be incredibly difficult for some people to do). The point is that we meet people where they are, provide a place to start, and then orient the process according to goals. Although folks may start with largely the same plan, they seldom finish in the same place. Some are high carb, some low . . . not surprisingly, some moderate. The one commonality these folks have—and it reflects the diets of non-Westernized populations—is the bulk of the food is whole and largely unprocessed. Nutrient density increases while total caloric intake decreases.

What's the goal of this? Today, we live in a world that is far removed from our hunter-gatherer ancestors. Some people liken our modern environment to an unnatural, zoo-like setting. We work long hours, mostly sitting down under fluorescent lights, with long commutes in gas-guzzling cars to come home to our toxic dwellings,

* The term nutrivore was first coined (to our knowledge) by Sarah Ballantyne.

wrapped in plastic siding and covered in wall-to-wall laminate, to watch a box of flickering images telling us why we want the next cool gadget and how such and such convenient food will save us so much time in the kitchen and has "a taste kids love." We exercise indoors on a hamster wheel–like contraption while watching more flickering images of how our bodies should be looking. The toxic pollution we breathe in, the chemicals that surround us in our homes, offices, and lawns, and pharmaceutical and recreational drugs and alcohol are foreign stressors to our bodies. We aren't sleeping enough and are addicted to caffeine to keep us going. We're in over our heads with mortgages, car loans, college debt, yet we've never before had such a high quality of living, compared to our ancestors. This challenge is intended to shake up your routine and help you find a nutritious and sustainable way of eating that will work for you.

BABY STEPS

This can be a BIG shift in eating for some of you who are new to the idea. If this all seems too overwhelming, we suggest considering the "baby step" protocol: eliminate all gluten and refined sugar from your diet for one full month (gluten-free whole grains, legumes, and full-fat dairy would still be allowed). This alone can result in amazing health benefits. After one month, transition your breakfast to Paleo for the next two weeks, then both breakfast and lunch become Paleo for the third and fourth weeks. Finally, start your thirty-day challenge of squeaky-clean 100 percent Paleo (no grains, legumes, dairy, or sweeteners). For other people, just eliminating all non-Paleo foods from the get-go is the best choice. Decide for yourself, and make it happen.

If you're ready to jump in with both feet, then the following challenge is a great tool to start making better choices for your body and for the planet.

A THIRTY-DAY "SUSTAINABLE NUTRIVORE" CHALLENGE

We're going to lay out a basic, thirty-day reset diet that will benefit most people and fits within a Whole30, Paleo, or real food template. This is not intended for individuals with eating disorders, for whom "everything in moderation" may actually be the best advice. For the rest of us, the advice of "everything in moderation" can often lead to overconsumption of hyperpalatable, ultraprocessed foods.

WHAT CAN I EAT?

Rather than focusing on what foods to avoid, we like to look at what you'll use to fill your plate over the next thirty days. Remember that prioritizing protein will help keep you feeling full!

Sustainable Proteins: Make sure you're getting enough high-quality protein from animals. As we laid out in the nutrition section, most people benefit from about twice the RDA of protein, which is about 1.6 grams of protein per kilogram of body weight.

To calculate your weight in kilograms, divide your body weight in pounds by 2.2 (there are also some great widgets online for this).

Then, multiply by 1.6 to get your personal RDA. As we've said, that's the bare minimum to avoid disease, so go ahead and multiply it by 2 again to aim for your protein goal.

You can look up how much protein your favorite foods contain, and here's a basic list of the protein content in common animal products, though both authors often eat larger portions than what's listed as "standard" 3.5-ounce servings:

Chicken, roasted	3.5oz	31g
Lamb, chops	3.5oz	22g
Beef, roasted	3.5oz	26g

Pork tenderloin	3.5oz	26g
Fish, cod	3.5oz	23g
Eggs, whole	2 eggs	14g
Cheese, cheddar	1oz	6.5g
Milk, whole	1 cup	8g

Eggs from pastured chickens are actually worth the extra money because their fats are significantly better than industrially raised chicken eggs; however, eggs are not as high in protein as you might think, at only six grams per egg. Sustainable, local fish and shellfish are awesome if you live near the coast, but there are some great frozen and canned options, too. Grass-fed, locally produced beef, lamb, goat, and pork are fantastic. Chicken and other poultry are actually not quite as nutrient dense nor as sustainable as larger herbivores and most wild fish because they are harder to source well. Game meats, like venison and elk, are excellent. Organ meats, such as liver, are very rich sources of vitamins and can be included in your diet on a weekly basis, and if you can't handle the strong taste, some folks like to freeze liver and then swallow the frozen pieces; there are some good sources of grass-fed liver capsules on our website.* Sausage and bacon are great, but be careful of what they add to the sausage—sometimes breadcrumbs are added to Irish sausages. Another common ingredient in sausages and other processed food is "hydrolyzed vegetable protein," which means gluten.

> While we feel that there are incredible benefits, both environmentally and for animal welfare, of sourcing well-managed, grass-finished beef, we also realize this may not be possible for everyone, at least not all of the time (just like eating 100

---

* For a deeper dive into protein and why animal products provide a more complete profile of the amino acids humans need, visit www.sacredcow.info/blog/are-all-proteins-created-equal.

percent organic produce is not realistic for everyone). In the nutrition chapter and elsewhere in the book, we've made the case that animal proteins are superior to plant proteins from a nutrient standpoint, and that increasing protein is generally a good idea for most. Beef finished in a feedlot can still be a better choice than a bagel or a twinkie. Buy the best quality food you can afford, but if it's not 100 percent pasture raised and organic, we still encourage you to eat a diet rich in animal proteins and produce.

Fat Sources: Foods that are good sources of fat include avocados, egg yolks (from pastured chickens), and fatty cuts of meat from pastured animals. To cook, use clarified butter,* ghee, tallow from grass-fed cows, bacon fat, and lard from pastured pork. Olive oil is great for salads and low-heat cooking, but saturated fat is ideal for high-heat cooking. Coconut oil is another fantastic saturated fat and a favorite among Paleo chefs, but it's not a locally produced item for most of us, so for sustainability reasons, you may want to limit its use.

Vegetables: Try to seek out locally grown, organic vegetables. In general, the darker the color, the more nutrient dense the vegetable is, but that's not to say that cauliflower and mushrooms aren't also great choices. Some of the most nutrient-dense vegetables include asparagus, broccoli, spinach, kale, watercress, sauerkraut, chard, and red bell peppers.

Fruits: Local, organic, seasonal fruit and berries are an ideal choice for treats, both nutritionally and when considering sustainability. If you're looking to lose weight, moderating your high-sugar fruit intake (like bananas, which probably don't grow near most of you!) is a good idea.

---

* See section on dairy.

Herbs and Spices: Fresh herbs like basil, cilantro, and fresh tarragon can definitely transform a meal, and most herbs are really nutrient dense. Seek out organic when possible.

Salt: Natural sea salt has the best profile of minerals. Surprisingly, though, sea salt has very little iodine. You can get some iodine from seaweed once a week or so. You can buy sheets of organic nori to use as wrappers for "sandwiches" and dulse or kelp flakes to sprinkle in soups and stews.

Nutrivore-Approved Condiments: Seek out condiments that don't contain added sugar (hello ketchup!) or industrially processed oils like canola. We both used to make our own mayo and dressing, but luckily today there are some great companies like Primal Kitchen, which has a full line of clean mayo (including a spicy version!), ketchup, salad dressings, and other condiments.

A NOTE ON CARBOHYDRATES IN GENERAL

We see many people avoiding roots and tubers while on a Paleo diet because they are trying to reduce their carbohydrate intake. Carbohydrates do have benefits such as lowering cortisol (stress), fueling highly glycemic workouts (like CrossFit), and acting like a prebiotic in your intestines (by feeding your good bacteria). Those with diabetes or other blood sugar regulation issues generally do better initially with lower carbohydrates, but some folks thrive on a higher intake of tuber-based starches and seasonal fruit. For this reason, we're not banning carbohydrate foods during the thirty days of your Nutrivore Challenge. Tinker and pay attention to how you feel, but avoid assuming what worked for one person is exactly what will work for you. The one "rule" is avoiding processed food.

LIMIT YOUR NUTS AND SEEDS

Although they are a really great source of nutrients, nuts and seeds are very calorically dense and easy to eat in excess, especially when salted. Also, the proper way to prepare raw nuts is to soak and then dehydrate them before eating, which few people have the time to do.

WHAT'S OFF THE MENU?

For the next thirty days, we recommend avoiding or strictly limiting your intake of the following:

Sweeteners: Avoid these for the next thirty days. Enjoy natural sweeteners like honey or maple syrup sparingly *after* your thirty-day challenge. Be careful of overconsuming sweetened things, even when they are marketed as "Paleo." Paleo cookies, muffins, and cakes are still cookies, muffins, and cakes and don't have a place in daily consumption. Please consider them occasional treats.

Condiments with Sugars and Additives: When shopping for condiments, avoid added sugars and impossible-to-pronounce chemical additives. These items should enhance your meal but not mask poor-quality ingredients. Watch out for hidden ingredients, like wheat in soy sauce (you can find coconut aminos at many natural grocery stores or online, which tastes like soy sauce).

Flours: There are many grain-free alternative flours out there, but be careful about re-creating hyperpalatable foods like brownies out of almond or coconut flour. We advise avoiding flours or making fancy desserts for your first thirty days and get used to classic techniques like stewing, baking, and grilling.

Grains and Legumes: For the thirty days of your challenge, avoid all grains and legumes (like quinoa, wheat, barley, lentils, and black beans). One big reason to avoid grains in general are because they're nutrient poor compared to organically grown roots and tubers. Also, people generally consume grains in the form of processed breads, pastas, cereals, and sweet foods. If you look at the nutrients contained in one cup of cooked hot whole-wheat cereal and compare it to one cup of baked sweet potato, sweet potatoes win the nutrient-density contest by a long shot. One cup of sweet potatoes contains 38,433 IU of vitamin A (769 percent of the daily value) in the form of beta-carotene, 39.2 milligrams of vitamin C (65 percent of the daily value), and is a very good source of the mineral manganese. What about the fiber? Sweet potatoes, and vegetables in general, are also a fantastic source of fiber.

The occasional consumption of properly prepared legumes and gluten-free grains may work for some folks on a health basis in the context of a Paleo diet template. However, environmentally speaking, grains are not an ideal crop. This is because, generally speaking, grains are grown using large-scale monocrop methods. Looking at sustainability, as well as the nutrition factors, it just doesn't add up for humans to be eating a grain-heavy diet. Legumes at least fix nitrogen and improve soil quality, and on our farm we do plant them as a cover crop to reduce soil erosion and increase soil nitrogen when a field is fallow.

Grains and legumes affect people differently. Some have clear gastrointestinal autoimmune reactions to gluten. Others get rashes, headaches, indigestion, or "brain fog." The truth is, they are not as nutrient dense as other sources of starches, such as roots and tubers, and actually contain antinutrients that can block absorption of vitamins and minerals. We've found most folks feel much better when they eliminate gluten and other grains from their diet. After your thirty-day Nutrivore Challenge, if you feel that you'd like to occasionally consume them, make them part of your 80-20 lifestyle, keeping them in the 20 percent. Record how you feel after reintroducing them and note any digestive or functional changes happening in your body after consumption.

Gluten, the protein in wheat, rye, and barley, is problematic not only for people like Diana with diagnosed celiac disease but also can cause a host of problems for many other people. Celiac symptoms can be silent; in fact, almost 50 percent of newly diagnosed celiac patients do not have regular GI distress. However, traditional testing for celiac only screens for antibodies to alpha-gliadin and transglutaminase-2, but there are multiple components that are not tested for, and which can cause reactions. This is why some people who have tested negative for celiac disease feel better when they are gluten-free. So, while you may be one of the people who feel little difference in your digestive system when you eat bread, gluten could still be wreaking havoc on your system and decreasing the absorption of nutrients.

Dairy: Ideally, you should pull out all dairy for your thirty-day Nutrivore Challenge. If you would like to reintroduce it after that period, record how you feel. In some people, dairy can cause acne or stuffiness, whereas in others digestive issues are the problem. Plain whole milk yogurt, crème fraîche, and raw-milk cheeses from grass-fed cows are a great source of fat-soluble vitamins and naturally occurring trans-fatty acids such as CLA (conjugated linoleic acid), which can help regulate glucose levels. Dairy is also a source of protein, although casein can be problematic in some people. So if dairy gives you a problem, don't eat it. American cheese and low-fat, fruit-flavored yogurts, however, are processed foods with poor nutrient density. Seek out full-fat grass-fed organic dairy whenever possible.

WHAT IF I DON'T EAT MEAT?

Believe it or not, we're not against people who choose not to eat meat out of personal preference. We've made the strong case that animal products are healthy and can be produced in an environmentally friendly way, and that avoiding them doesn't necessarily mean you're causing less harm in your diet. However, we get it, some people don't like the taste or, for whatever reason, don't wish to eat animal products. Plant-based proteins are much higher in calories and carbohydrates, and have fewer nutrients than meat. We highly encourage you to give meat a try, and have some resources available at Sacredcow.info for those "meat curious" and looking to incorporate some form of animal protein into their diets. If fish is all you can stomach, you can get fantastic protein and lots of nutrients from seafood, especially fatty fish like salmon or sardines and oysters or other shellfish. If animal flesh is completely off the table, shoot for eggs from pasture-raised chickens and fermented dairy products from grass-fed cows, like cheese and yogurt.

HOW MUCH TO EAT?

This is always the next question we get. Though some have had great luck with fasting, one meal a day, and other types of eating windows, if this is all new to you, a great starting point is the following:

3 meals a day

Protein: the size of your palm, about 4-8 ounces, depending on your size and need

Nonstarchy vegetables: piled high on your plate

Starchy vegetables: athletes, the equivalent of about two small/medium sweet potatoes a day; nonathletes should start with about one.

1 tablespoon or so of healthy fat (salad dressing, butter, avocado)

Snacks: if necessary, have a handful (not a 5lb bag), of nuts and a piece of fruit

OK, THAT'S ALL GREAT, SO REALLY, WHAT DO I ACTUALLY EAT?

Have you ever had scrambled eggs and fruit for breakfast, a big salad for lunch with some grilled fish, and a steak and some broccoli for dinner? Then you've already eaten the way we're prescribing!

Some find making a meal matrix, like Robb first developed in his book *The Paleo Solution*, quite helpful. Make a list of ten meats, ten veggies, ten fats, ten herbs and spices, and ten other components like fruits and nuts. If you take one item from each of these columns, combine them and consider that a meal, you have ten thousand meal options. If that was one meal a day, you would potentially not see the same meal for *twenty-seven years*. By focusing on what you can eat and not what you're removing, the opportunities for meals are virtually endless. Here's a sample:

NUTRIVORE MEAL MATRIX

Make a list of ten meats, ten veggies, ten fats, ten herbs and spices, and ten other components like fruits and nuts. If you take one item from each of these columns, combine them and consider that a meal, **you have ten thousand meal options**. If that was one meal a day, you would potentially not see the same meal for **twenty-seven years**.

MEATS & PROTEINS	VEGGIES	FATS	HERBS & SPICES	OTHER
Grass-fed, pastured, wild	Seasonal/organic	Pasture-raised or organic	Organic	Organic
Steak*	Broccoli*	Butter	Basil*	Nori*
Salmon*	Carrots	Olive oil	Rosemary*	Pumpkin seeds*
Chicken	Spinach*	Coconut oil	Chili powder	Brazil nuts*
Lamb chops*	Asparagus*	Avocado	Turmeric*	Blueberries*
Ground pork*	Bok choy*	Avocado oil	Cilantro*	Raspberries*
Eggs*	String beans	Tallow	Sage	Cantaloupe*
Liver/organ meats*	Kale*	Ghee	Parsley*	Kimchee*
Sardines*	Cauliflower*	Coconut milk	Red pepper flakes	Sauerkraut*
Ground beef*	Green peas*	Bacon	Cumin	Mushrooms*
Oysters*	Onion/garlic/leeks*	Lard	Thyme*	Cherries*

* indicates foods that are particularly micronutrient dense

WHAT DOES THIS LOOK LIKE?

You might be wondering what a day of food could look like eating this way.

This is a typical day for Diana. "I often eat eggs for breakfast with some sort of vegetable from the farm. Lunch is frequently a salad with some tuna or salmon, and dinner is whatever meat is thawed in the fridge, plus whatever veggies are on hand."

Breakfast: 3 pasture-raised eggs in an omelet with organic spinach and a side of fresh/frozen organic berries.

Lunch: Big salad filled with colorful vegetables like peppers, carrots, tomatoes, cucumbers, topped with some pumpkin seeds for crunch and a 4–6 ounce piece of wild salmon.

Dinner: 4–6 ounce grass-fed steak with a sweet potato and roasted broccoli.

And this is a typical day for Robb. "I tend to eat on the low-carb side of things, but that varies with the seasons. In the summer I eat a fair amount of fruit. In the winter you will see more root veggies. Given my work schedule and two young daughters, I try to simplify both cooking and meals, so breakfast or lunch is almost always leftovers from the previous evening dinner. Today is a pretty good example."

Breakfast: Tri-tip reheated, bowl of mixed berries and coconut flakes, homemade sauerkraut.

Lunch: Huge salad with wild canned salmon, lettuce, tomatoes, avocados, carrots, and green onions.

Dinner: Skirt steak, large artichokes, baked sweet potatoes with cinnamon and grass-fed butter.

(The girls and I "might" have shared some 85 percent dark chocolate for dessert.)

BUT WHAT ABOUT THOSE OTHER "HEALTHY" DIETS?

Let's take a look at what a typical breakfast would be on a variety of what *US News & World Report* continually ranks as the best diets. Maybe you'd like to do an experiment and see how full you are eating each of these breakfasts. When would you be ready for lunch in each of these scenarios? Which meal do you think packs the best nutrient density? Which of these diets is based on monocrop agriculture?

Compared to the nutrivore breakfast, these other examples are low in fat, low in protein, and high in carbs. Eating this way in a fasted state (first thing in the morning) can set a person up for a blood sugar roller coaster. The DASH diet, which has been highly promoted by mainstream dietitians and the media, is particularly appalling: cereal, toast with margarine, and orange juice! Who eats margarine still? Didn't it disappear along with Aqua Net in the 1980s? And we all know orange juice is just sugar, right? There are way better sources of vitamin C than orange juice.

And let's look at the macrobiotic diet. It starts the day with *no* fat at all (and most of these other diets are pretty low fat in our opinion). The oatmeal has 12 grams of protein but 64 grams of carbs, 2 slices of whole wheat bread adds another 8 grams of protein and 26 grams of carbs, and apple butter adds another 14 grams of carbs (and nothing else as far as vitamins or minerals)—that's a total of 104 grams of carbs (more than I eat in a whole day) with 20 grams of incomplete protein and no fat to slow digestion down. It's hard to see how one could make it to lunch without passing out! All this skim milk and toast (with margarine) is definitely not more nutrient dense (nor more sustainable) than the real-food breakfast shown for the nutrivore.*

---

* For a deeper dive on micronutrient content comparisons on meat-rich, nutrient-dense omnivore, and vegan diets, please visit www.sacredcow.info/blog/what-if-we-all-went-plant-based.

WHICH BREAKFAST DO YOU THINK IS HEALTHIEST?

Dash Diet
¾ cup bran flakes cereal
(¾ cup shredded wheat cereal) with 1 medium banana and 1 cup low-fat milk
1 slice whole wheat bread with 1 teaspoon unsalted margarine
1 cup orange juice

Weight Watchers
1 slice of whole wheat bread
1 tablespoon of peanut butter
1 small banana
1 cup strawberries

Mayo Clinic Diet
1 cup whole-grain breakfast cereal
1 cup skim milk
1 medium orange
Calorie-free beverage

Acid Alkaline Diet
1½ egg whites
½ tablespoon soy milk
Dash black pepper
Dash garlic powder
⅛ teaspoon sea salt
2 asparagus spears, chopped
½ tablespoon clarified butter

TLC Diet
1 cup oatmeal with 1 cup fat-free milk and ¼ cup raisins
1 cup honeydew melon
1 cup calcium-fortified orange juice
1 cup coffee (with 2 tablespoons fat-free milk)

Flexitarian Diet
1 slice whole-grain bread
1½ tablespoons almond butter or peanut butter
1 sliced apple

Macrobiotic Diet
2 cups oatmeal
2 slices whole wheat sourdough bread with 2 tablespoons apple butter
Green tea

Sustainable Nutrivore Diet
3 eggs
¼ onion, chopped
½ cup chopped tomato
4½ ounces baby spinach
1 cup blueberries
½ avocado
(Ideally, pasture-raised eggs; substitute equivalent amounts of other seasonal vegetables and fruits)

OTHER CONSIDERATIONS

Just because a food is considered OK for the nutrivore diet doesn't mean that you are free to eat ten pounds of bacon at each meal, or chase each snack with a gallon of coconut milk. Athletes should naturally consume more starchy vegetables like roots (carrots and parsnips) and tubers (potatoes and sweet potatoes). The macronutrient combination and calorie load that works for a twenty-five-year-old athlete may not work for a fifty-year-old recovering from hip surgery. It's best to consider your weight loss goals, stress level, and activity level. For weight loss, consider consuming the bulk of your daily starch intake in a post-workout meal. More active people can include more starches. Winter squashes like butternut are lower in calories than potatoes or sweet potatoes.

DON'T EAT FOR WINTER!

We're both huge fans of Marty Kendall's work on nutrient density (more on Sacredcow.info about that), and he brought to our attention the work of Cian Foley, who is a champion of the Don't Eat for Winter diet. The idea is that carbs alone or fat alone are not necessarily going to spark overeating. However, the magical combination of carbs plus fat seems to be an unnaturally winning combination to our brain's circuits. Most hyperpalatable junk food is this combo—think about potato chips. It's hard to overeat plain boiled potatoes, but fry them in a vat of oil and many people can crush a whole bag in one sitting.

Some of the most hyperpalatable foods include mashed potatoes (with butter), chocolate chips, potato chips, custard, French toast, waffles, blueberry muffins, hash browns, garlic bread, and human breast milk.

WATCH YOUR OMEGA-3s AND OMEGA-6s

The typical American diet tends to contain fourteen to twenty-five times more omega-6 fatty acids than omega-3 fatty acids. One cup of whole wheat flour has a 20:1 ratio of omega-6 to omega-3. One cup of cooked long-grain white rice is better, at 4:1. Soybean oil has a 7:1 ratio of omega 6:3. Compare this to kale, with a 1:1 ratio, or coho salmon, which has a 1:7 ratio (seven times more omega-3 than omega-6), and you can see where the healthy choices are. As we mentioned in the nutrition section, grass-fed beef does have more omega-3s in general, but it's not a fantastic source of omega-3s. Your best bet to improve your ratio of omega-3 to -6 is to remove foods with lots of omega-6 from your diet (generally this means highly processed foods) and eat a diet that is filled with lots of seafood and vegetables.

FOCUS ON MICRONUTRIENTS

You shouldn't feel hungry, but it's also not ideal to eat past capacity. Tracking your total calories can be very helpful for some folks who have noticed weight gain. Sometimes, eating a nutrient-dense diet can mean you're overconsuming calories. Trying to get all your micronutrients from food is a fun challenge and really helps you understand the importance of prioritizing animal protein, plus how increasing your intake of brightly colored vegetables can help you meet these goals. While some foods may seem nutrient dense by calorie, it's important to take into account the serving size.

A NOTE ON MEAL TIMING

Try to shut down the kitchen by about 7:00 PM or even earlier. Studies show that late-night eating is more likely to lead to weight gain, and that front-loading your calories is a good idea. The idea is "breakfast like a king, lunch like a prince, dinner like a pauper," which seems to be the opposite of how many Americans eat. Although there are tons of bloggers "crushing it" with fasting protocols, for someone just entering into this way of eating, we feel that there's no need to skip meals during this thirty-day intro phase—just focus on three meals per day, making sure you load up on protein early in the day. Everyone is unique, so please tinker with your own diet until you find a good ratio that works for you.

CLEAN OUT THE PANTRY

Before you begin the thirty-day challenge, get rid of everything ultraprocessed in your kitchen. You may be feeling guilty about that box of bow tie pasta on the back shelf, but trust us, you don't need it. The condiments in your fridge likely contain canola oil or added sugars. Clean out everything that is ultraprocessed and put it in a box and donate what's not expired or opened. If you live with folks who aren't doing this challenge, fill a special cabinet drawer with the "off-plan" foods so they're not right there in front of you, calling your name every time you open the main cabinet.

TRACK YOUR INTAKE

Using meal-tracking software, even for only a few days, can help you know how many calories, protein, fat, and carbs you're eating, and if you're even close to meeting your micronutrient goals. For these reasons, Cronometer is a great tool. You can set up a free account and visit our website, Sacredcow.info, for a tutorial on how to customize your settings. We also have some great tools to help you discover how to best optimize your diet and links to organizations that run nutrition boot camps and nutrient-density challenges.

SEE HOW YOU FEEL

Notice how you're sleeping, if your little aches and pains are fading away, if you feel more mental clarity, better skin, improved mood, and so on. There are so many benefits to eating well that are beyond just a change in weight. The Whole30 diet has done a great job of having folks focus on "nonscale victories," and their website has some great resources. During the thirty days of the challenge, we recommend that you record how you feel, how you're sleeping, what you're eating, and which symptoms you're experiencing so that you can start to notice patterns. It also helps to keep you on track!

AFTER THIRTY DAYS

Take a look at your Nutrivore Challenge journal and note what shifted for you. Did you have more energy? How did your food prep and buying patterns change? Did you connect with a local farmer and fill your freezer with better meat? Did your skin improve, or did those joint pains you used to feel when you first got up go away?

How you incorporate this new way of eating into the rest of your life is a personal choice, but if you want to be less restrictive with your diet, taking two meals of the week (assuming you're eating three meals a day, seven days a week) should help you still do your best from a nutrient-density perspective yet allow for the occasional "kick your heels up" social occasion. Others shoot for an 80-20 approach, or keep it pretty on plan except for holidays. It's really up to you and what works for your lifestyle and budget. We both tend to eat this way most of the time but travel frequently and realize that it's not always easy to be "squeaky clean" 100 percent of the time. That's OK. From a nutrient-density and sustainability perspective, a typical steak may be the best option on the menu at an Italian restaurant where the other choices are pasta or chicken. Just because it's a plant, doesn't mean that it's a healthier or more sustainable choice. Do what's best in your current situation, keep your home as healthy and sustainable as possible, and cook most of your meals yourself. Avoid excess drinking and desserts and prioritize protein.

IN CLOSING

We recognize this was a lot to take in, and appreciate your sticking with us. We hope we've shed some light on why meat has been unfairly maligned, the importance of animals to humans as a food source, how it can be produced in a regenerative way, and why a food system without animals may actually cause more harm than good. Although we admittedly have some biases (who doesn't?), it is our goal to actually address the topic as thoroughly as possible, as getting this story right (or wrong) will affect the lives of billions of people. As Joseph Stalin cynically (but accurately) observed, "A single death is a tragedy, a million a statistic." Although our hope is that this work will find broad applications, and literally "help the world," both authors have young children that will live through what may be the most challenging time in human history. Neither of us want to go to our graves knowing we left our children a disaster.

The diet plan we've presented comes from years of clinical work and feedback from hundreds of thousands of people who have regenerated their own health through changing the food they eat. We have developed Sacredcow.info as a place to continue the conversation and provide additional resources and new research in the field of sustainable and regenerative food systems. You'll also find videos from health experts and farmers changing the food system.

THE SYSTEM NEEDS TO CHANGE

The fact is, we can't afford *not* to change how we are growing food and how we are eating. **We're overweight, metabolically broken, our small towns are dying, and we're ruining our soil.** Some complain that there's not enough peer-reviewed research backing up the type of system we're advocating for, but we know of many farmers changing over to regenerative agriculture and saving their farms and their health. Many of these regenerative pioneers are featured in the film *Sacred Cow*.

We're also seeing more creative direct-to-consumer marketing by farmers. By cutting out the middle man and selling directly to consumers, farmers can make a much better living. One thing people don't realize about highly processed meat substitutes and lab meats is that the ones benefiting from this are the large food manufacturers. It's convenient for their profits that the marketing story is about saving animal suffering, improving human health, and being better for the environment. But don't be fooled. The main driver behind these products is profit.

Remember, cattle can consume crop residues and other plant matter that we humans can't digest on land we can't crop while increasing ecosystem health.

WHAT IS THE FUTURE OF FOOD?

We're at a critical point right now where we can turn things around or we can ensure the human population won't succeed. Would it be absolutely crazy to suggest that we deemphasize global chemical monocropping and pay more attention to soil health, water use, and nutrient-rich food instead of human "feed"? When considering the global food systems, could it make more sense to emphasize regional reliance while leveraging the power of central distribution when and where it makes sense?

It's basic human nature to create us-versus-them scenarios and to project our fears onto objects other than the real problems. It's time we realize that governments, multinational corporations, and the media all benefit from our current food system and food tribe infighting. The problem is that, we, as humans, don't. When we fight about different facets of what the ideal diet is, big food wins every time.

The real threat to human health and the planet is industrially produced food. We should *all* agree on this and find a way to move forward, allowing people to choose which version of a real food diet works best for their bodies.

Given the complexity (and importance) of the topics covered in this book, it would be nice to leave you with a sense of inspiration, perhaps even excitement. The world can look pretty bleak at times. The following may not fit the bill for "excitement," but we hope that it at least sows the seed of curiosity:

The challenges we face globally, from the health of people to the diversity (of both organisms and ideas) and stability of the planet, are often portrayed as a predicament rather than a problem. A problem suggests some kind of solution. The work to implement the solution may be challenging, but there is the proverbial "light at the end of the tunnel." A predicament, by contrast, suggests, at best, perhaps choosing one of a variety of poor options. The current row-crop-centric food system is indeed a predicament. Not only is it unsustainable from an ecological perspective; it is poised to bankrupt the economies of developed nations thanks to the exponentially increasing health-care costs of a broken system built on processed foods. These are nontrivial considerations, as an inability or unwillingness to properly address our challenges could at best result in incredible suffering from economic and health challenges, but could also realistically represent an existential threat not just to humanity but to our neighboring species in this world. That's clearly a big deal, but there is something about all this that is less immediately tangible but perhaps more important than extinction—our freedom and our souls.

IN CLOSING

The row-crop-centric food system proposed and embraced by academia, media, and government is now, and will be, owned by a few gargantuan multinational corporations. These all-powerful entities will control every feature of our lives by controlling the molecular basis of our lives: food. People who live in Ecuador will feel the pressure of rich bureaucrats in Europe and the US who have decided "what is best for everyone." We'd like to again suggest that we embrace the concept of food sovereignty, allowing regional food systems to flourish. Some may dismiss these ideas as dystopian ramblings, but others may recognize that a fair amount of roadway has already been paved toward this Brave New World.

We know we said that we want to leave you with a sense of empowerment and excitement . . . Here it is: we do not face a predicament; we face a problem. The problem is not technological, moral, or even genetic (although some hardwired human tendencies do pose challenges in all this). Our problem is one of perspective. If there is a human failing, perhaps more dangerous than any other, it is the predilection toward superficial, black-and-white, good-versus-bad simplifications of processes that are infinitely complex. We convince ourselves we can control the world when in fact our best effort, and only real hope, is to act as stewards. We need to shift from seeing ourselves as separate from and above nature to seeing ourselves as beings participating with and loving our planet—not just because of what it can provide to us, but because the world in itself is magnificent and complex. Humanity cannot defy the laws of nature, but we are also different from any other organism because we CAN change our perspective. It has been the iterative process of perceptual shifts that has brought us to our current challenges and opportunities. Our way forward will be defined by what perspective we choose to embrace.

ACKNOWLEDGMENTS

Thank you to those of you who believed in our message and supported our work and the film. We're certain that there are many names we're forgetting at the time of writing this, so we apologize in advance to those who have helped along the way whom we've missed in this list.

Thank you to Chris Kresser for doing much of the research on Mormon longevity and micronutrients, and Alex Leif for helping with the research into grass-fed versus typical beef, and the work of Zoe Harcombe, Belinda Fettke, Frédéric Leroy, Marty Kendall, Tyler Cartwright, Luis Villaseñor, Melissa Urban, Bill Lagakos, Dr. Drew Ramsey, Dr. Mark Hyman, Mark Sisson, Dr. Georgia Ede, and Adele Hite, who all helped or inspired the nutrition section.

We also had help and inspiration on the environmental section from Andrew Rodgers, Jason Rowntree, Russ Conser, Nicolette Hahn Niman, Peter Ballerstedt, Judith Schwartz, Sara Place, Charles Massey, Bobby Gil, Allan Savory, Frank Mitloehner, Jim Howell, and Joel Salatin.

The ethics section was influenced by the incredible work of Frédéric Leroy, Belinda Fettke, Lierre Keith, and Andrew Smith.

Many thanks to the talented James Cooper for cover design and graphics; he has been an absolute pleasure to work with. Thanks also go to Diana's advisory and support team of James Connolly,

ACKNOWLEDGMENTS

Abby Fuller, Meg Chatham, Lauren Stine, Rachel James, and Magnus Eriksson.

Special thanks from Diana: I would like to send special thanks to my husband, Andrew, my Dad, my two amazing kids, Anson and Phoebe, Janet and Gil Rodgers, and my friends Kirsty Allore, Tallie Katwinkle, Michelle Tam, Kristin Canty, Emily Deans, and especially James Connolly, for all of your support, to the ladies on the farm crew, MaryLiz and Meredith, and to Marjie Findlay and Geoff Freeman at Clark Farm. Also, thank you to Robb for helping to make the book a reality.

Special thanks from Robb: I'd like to thank my coauthor Diana Rodgers for showing nearly superhuman tenacity in this and the related film project. The message we have to share is one of nuance, and does not jibe well with the human tendency for extremism and binary solutions. Few will know how hard she has fought and how much she has sacrificed to bring this book to life.

I'd be a terrible husband and father if I did not say thank you to my wife, Nicki, and my daughters, Zoe and Sagan. There were many dinners I could not cook and games of "wrestle-fight" I could not take part in while working on this book.

A final thanks goes out to the folks who have given my musings a shot. My goal has always been to leave the world a better place, and I can only do that if I positively influence the people around me.

NOTES

CHAPTER 1: MEAT AS SCAPEGOAT

1   Francisco Sánchez-Bayo and Kris A.G. Wyckhuys, "Worldwide Decline of the Entomofauna: A Review of Its Drivers," *Biological Conservation* 232 (April 2019): 8–27, www.sciencedirect.com/science/article/abs/pii/S0006320718313636.

2   Gerardo Ceballos et al., "Accelerated Modern Human-Induced Species Losses: Entering the Sixth Mass Extinction," *Science Advances* 1, no. 5 (June 19, 2015), advances.sciencemag.org/content/1/5/e1400253.full.

3   Sánchez-Bayo and Wyckhuys, "Worldwide Decline," 8–27.

4   "The Cost of Diabetes," American Diabetes Association, accessed December 30, 2019, www.diabetes.org/resources/statistics/cost-diabetes.

5   "Adult Obesity Causes & Consequences," Overweight & Obesity, Centers for Disease Control and Prevention, accessed December 30, 2019, https://www.cdc.gov/obesity/adult/causes.html.

6   Bjørn Lomborg, "Ban the Beef?" Project Syndicate, November 21, 2018, www.project-syndicate.org/commentary/meat-production-overstated-effect-on-climate-change-by-bjorn-lomborg-2018-11.

7   Frédéric Leroy, "Chapter Eight – Meat as a *Pharmakon*: An Exploration of the Biosocial Complexities of Meat Consumption," *Advances in Food and Nutrition Research* 87 (2019): 409–446, doi.org/10.1016/bs.afnr.2018.07.002.

8   Jeffrey Kluger, "Sorry Vegans: Here's How Meat-Eating Made Us Human," *Time*, March 9, 2016, time.com/4252373/meat-eating-veganism-evolution.

9   Katherine D. Zink and Daniel E. Lieberman, "Impact of Meat and Lower Paleolithic Food Processing Techniques on Chewing in Humans," *Nature* 531 (2016): 500–3, www.nature.com/articles/nature16990.

10 Jacques Peretti, "Why Our Food Is Making Us Fat," *The Guardian*, June 11, 2012, www.theguardian.com/business/2012/jun/11/why-our-food-is-making-us-fat.

11   Table 1 in "Summary Report of the EAT-*Lancet* Commission," EAT, January 16, 2019, eatforum.org/content/uploads/2019/07/EAT-Lancet_Commission_Summary_Report.pdf.

CHAPTER 2: ARE HUMANS OMNIVORES?

1   Leslie C. Aiello and Peter Wheeler, "The Expensive-Tissue Hypothesis: The Brain and the Digestive System in Human and Primate Evolution," *Current Anthropology* 36, no. 2 (April 1995): 199–221, doi.org/10.1086/204350.

2   George J. Armelagos, "Brain Evolution, the Determinates of Food Choice, and the Omnivore's Dilemma," *Critical Reviews in Food Science and Nutrition* 54, no. 10 (2014): 1330–41, doi.org/10.1080/10408398.2011.635817.

3   Francesca Luca, George H. Perry, and Anna Di Rienzo, "Evolutionary Adaptations to Dietary Changes," *Annual Review of Nutrition* 30 (August 21, 2010): 291–314, www.ncbi.nlm.nih.gov/pmc/articles/PMC4163920.

4   Loren Cordain et al., "Plant-Animal Subsistence Ratios and Macronutrient Energy Estimations in Worldwide Hunter-Gatherer Diets," *American Journal of Clinical Nutrition* 71, no. 3 (March 2000): 682–92, academic.oup.com/ajcn/article/71/3/682/4729121.

5   Michael Gurven and Hillard Kaplan, "Longevity Among Hunter-Gatherers: A Cross-Cultural Examination," *Population and Development Review* 33, no. 2 (June 2007): 321–65; Vybarr Cregan-Reid, "Hunter-Gatherers Live Nearly as Long as We Do but with Limited Access to Healthcare," The Conversation, October 31, 2018, theconversation.com/hunter-gatherers-live-nearly-as-long-as-we-do-but-with-limited-access-to-healthcare-104157.

6   Hillard Kaplan et al., "Coronary Atherosclerosis in Indigenous South American Tsimane: A Cross-Sectional Cohort Study," *The Lancet* 398, no. 10080 (April 29, 2017): 1730–39, https://www.thelancet.com/journals/lancet/article/PIIS0140-6736(17)30752-3/fulltext; Herman Pontzer, Brian M. Wood, and David A. Reichlen, "Hunter-Gatherers as Models in Public Health," *Obesity Reviews* (December 3, 2018), www.ncbi.nlm.nih.gov/pubmed/30511505; James H. O'Keefe Jr. and Loren Cordain, "Cardiovascular Disease Resulting from a Diet and Lifestyle at Odds with Our Paleolithic Genome: How to Become a 21st-Century Hunter-Gatherer," *Mayo Clinic Proceedings* 79, no. 1 (January 2004): 101–8, www.mayoclinicproceedings.org/article/S0025-6196(11)63262-X/fulltext.

CHAPTER 3: ARE WE EATING TOO MUCH MEAT?

1   Gregory S. Okin, "Environmental Impacts of Food Consumption by Dogs and Cats," *PLOS One* (August 2, 2017), journals.plos.org/plosone/article?id=10.1371/journal.pone.0181301.

2   "The Changing American Diet: A Report Card," Center for Science in the Public Interest, September 23, 2013, cspinet.org/resource/changing-american-diet.

NOTES

3   Robert R. Wolfe, "The Role of Dietary Protein in Optimizing Muscle Mass, Function and Health Outcomes in Older Individuals," *British Journal of Nutrition* 108, no. S2 (August 2012): S88–S93, doi.org/10.1017/S0007114512002590.

4   "Body Measurements," Centers for Disease Control and Prevention, July 15, 2016, www.cdc.gov/nchs/fastats/body-measurements.htm.

5   "Dietary Reference Intakes Tables and Application," National Academies of Sciences, Engineering, and Medicine, accessed December 30, 2019. nationalacademies.org/hmd/Activities/Nutrition/SummaryDRIs/DRI-Tables.aspx.

6   Institute of Medicine, *Dietary Reference Intakes: For Energy Carbohydrate, Fiber, Fat, Fatty Acids, Cholesterol, Protein, and Amino Acids* (Washington, DC: National Academies Press, 2005).

7   David McCay, *Protein Element in Nutrition* (London: Longmans, Green, 1912).

8   "Dietary Reference Intakes: Macronutrients."

9   J. L. Krok-Schoen et al., "Low Dietary Protein Intakes and Associated Dietary Patterns and Functional Limitations in an Aging Population: A NHANES Analysis," *Journal of Nutrition, Health & Aging* 23 (2019), link.springer.com/article/10.1007/s12603-019-1174-1.

10 Jean-Philippe Bonjour, "Nutritional Disturbance in Acid–Base Balance and Osteoporosis: A Hypothesis That Disregards the Essential Homeostatic Role of the Kidney," *British Journal of Nutrition* 110, no. 7 (October 14, 2013): 1168–77, doi.org/10.1017/S000711451300096291-3-31.

11 Jose Antonio et al., "A High Protein Diet Has No Harmful Effects: A One-Year Crossover Study in Resistance-Trained Males," *Journal of Nutrition and Metabolism* 2016 (2016): 1–5, www.ncbi.nlm.nih.gov/pubmed/27807480.

12 William F. Martin, Lawrence E. Armstrong, and Nancy R. Rodriguez, "Dietary Protein Intake and Renal Function," *Nutrition & Metabolism* 2, no. 25 (September 20, 2005), nutritionandmetabolism.biomedcentral.com/articles/10.1186/1743-7075-2-25.

13 Margriet S. Westerterp-Plantenga, Sofie G. Lemmens, and Klaas R. Westerterp, "Dietary Protein—Its Role in Satiety, Energetics, Weight Loss and Health," *British Journal of Nutrition* 108, no. S2 (2012), www.ncbi.nlm.nih.gov/pubmed/23107521.

14 Sigal Sviri et al., "Vitamin B12 and Mortality in Critically Ill," *Diet and Nutrition in Critical Care* (2016): 973–82, link.springer.com/referenceworkentry/10.1007%2F978-1-4614-7836-2_45; Christel Chalouhi et al., "Neurological Consequences of Vitamin B12 Deficiency and Its Treatment," *Pediatric Emergency Care* 24, no. 8 (2008): 538–41, insights.ovid.com/crossref?an=00006565-200808000-00007.

15 S. H. A. Holt, Jennie C. Brand-Miller, Peter Petocz, and E. Farmakalidis, "A Satiety Index of Common Foods," *European Journal of Clinical Nutrition* 49, no. 9 (1995): 627–90, www.researchgate.net/publication/15701207_A_Satiety_Index_of_common_foods.

16 David S. Weigle et al., "A High-Protein Diet Induces Sustained Reductions in Appetite, Ad Libitum Caloric Intake, and Body Weight Despite Compensatory Changes in Diurnal Plasma Leptin and Ghrelin Concentrations," *American*

Journal of Clinical Nutrition 82, no.1 (July 2005): 41–48, academic.oup.com/ajcn/article/82/1/41/4863422.

17 Jia-Yi Dong et al., "Effects of High-Protein Diets on Body Weight, Glycaemic Control, Blood Lipids and Blood Pressure in Type 2 Diabetes: Meta-analysis of Randomised Controlled Trials," *British Journal of Nutrition* 110, no. 5 (2013): 781–89, www.cambridge.org/core/journals/british-journal-of-nutrition/article/effects-of-highprotein-diets-on-body-weight-glycaemic-control-blood-lipids-and-blood-pressure-in-type-2-diabetes-metaanalysis-of-randomised-controlled-trials/4D4F7A3943BE752FB061CE60671204B1.

18 Kelly A. Meckling, Caitriona O'Sullivan, and Dayna Saari, "Comparison of a Low-Fat Diet to a Low-Carbohydrate Diet on Weight Loss, Body Composition, and Risk Factors for Diabetes and Cardiovascular Disease in Free-Living, Overweight Men and Women," *Journal of Clinical Endocrinology & Metabolism* 89, no. 6 (June 1, 2004): 2717–23, academic.oup.com/jcem/article/89/6/2717/2870310.

19 Andreas Wittke et al., "Protein Supplementation to Augment the Effects of High Intensity Resistance Training in Untrained Middle-Aged Males: The Randomized Contolled PUSH Trial," *BioMed Research International* 2017, www.hindawi.com/journals/bmri/2017/3619398.

20 Sophie Miquel-Kergoat et al., "Effects of Chewing on Appetite, Food Intake and Gut Hormones: A Systematic Review and Meta-analysis," *Physiology & Behavior* 151 (November 1, 2015): 88–96, www.sciencedirect.com/science/article/pii/S0031938415300317.

21 "Global Meat-Eating Is on the Rise, Bringing Surprising Benefits," *Economist*, May 4, 2019, www.economist.com/international/2019/05/04/global-meat-eating-is-on-the-rise-bringing-surprising-benefits; Charlotte G. Neumann et al., "Meat Supplementation Improves Growth, Cognitive, and Behavioral Outcomes in Kenyan Children," *Journal of Nutrition* 137 no. 4 (April 2007): 1119–23, ncbi.nlm.nih.gov/pubmed/17374691.

CHAPTER 4: DOES MEAT CAUSE CHRONIC DISEASE?

1 Bradley C. Johnston et al., "Unprocessed Red Meat and Processed Meat Consumption: Dietary Guideline Recommendations from the Nutritional Recommendations (NutriRECS) Consortium," *Annals of Internal Medicine* (November 19, 2019), https://annals.org/aim/fullarticle/2752328/unprocessed-red-meat-processed-meat-consumption-dietary-guideline-recommendations-from.

2 Rita Rubin, "Backlash over Meat Dietary Recommendations Raises Questions About Corporate Ties to Nutrition Scientists," *JAMA* 323, no. 2 (January 15, 2020): 401–404, doi.org/10.1001/jama.2019.21441.

3 John P.A. Ioannidis, "Why Most Published Research Findings Are False," *PLoS Medicine* 2 no. 8 (August 30, 2005): e124, doi.org/10.1371/journal.pmed.0020124.

4 Jonathan D. Schoenfeld and John P.A. Ioannidis, "Is Everything We Eat Associated with Cancer? A Systematic Cookbook Review," *American Journal of Clinical Nutrition* 97 no. 1 (January 2013): 127–134, doi.org/10.3945/ajcn.112.047142.

NOTES

5   Geoffrey C. Marks, Maria Celia Hughes, Jolieke C. van der Pols, "Relative Validity of Food Intake Estimates Using a Food Frequency Questionnaire Is Associated with Sex, Age, and Other Personal Characteristics," *Journal of Nutrition* 136, no. 2 (February 2006): 459–65, academic.oup.com/jn/article/136/2/459/4743763.

6   M. Fogelholm, N. Kanerva, and S. Männistö, "Association Between Red and Processed Meat Consumption and Chronic Diseases: The Confounding Role of Other Dietary Factors," *European Journal of Clinical Nutrition* 69 (2015): 1060–65, www.ncbi.nlm.nih.gov/pubmed/25969395.

7   Nicola Davis, "Is Sugar Really as Addictive as Cocaine? Scientists Row over Effect on Body and Brain," *Guardian*, August 26, 2017, www.theguardian.com/society/2017/aug/25/is-sugar-really-as-addictive-as-cocaine-scientists-row-over-effect-on-body-and-brain.

8   Cheryl D. Fryar, Margaret D. Carroll, and Cynthia L. Ogden, "Prevalence of Overweight, Obesity, and Severe Obesity Among Adults Aged 20 and Over: United States, 1960–1962 Through 2015–2016," Centers for Disease Control and Prevention, updated October 16, 2018, www.cdc.gov/nchs/data/hestat/obesity_adult_15_16/obesity_adult_15_16.htm; Eric A. Finkelstein et al., "Obesity and Severe Obesity Forecasts Through 2030," *American Journal of Preventive Medicine* 42, no. 6 (June 2012): 563–70, www.ajpmonline.org/article/S0749-3797%2812%2900146-8/fulltext.

9   Michelle R. van Dellen, J. C. Isherwood, and J. E. Delose, "How Do People Define Moderation?" *Appetite* 101 (June 2016): 156–62, www.ncbi.nlm.nih.gov/pubmed/26964691.

10 Eric W. Manheimer et al., "Paleolithic Nutrition for Metabolic Syndrome: Systematic Review and Meta-analysis," *American Journal of Clinical Nutrition* 102, no. 4 (October 2015): 922–32, www.ncbi.nlm.nih.gov/pmc/articles/PMC4588744; Brittanie Chester et al., "The Effects of Popular Diets on Type 2 Diabetes Management," *Diabetes Metabolism Research and Reviews* (May 23, 2019), www.ncbi.nlm.nih.gov/pubmed/31121637; Hana Kahleova et al., "A Plant-Based Diet in Overweight Individuals in a 16-Week Randomized Clinical Trial: Metabolic Benefits of Plant Protein," *Nutrition & Diabetes* 8, no. 58 (2018), www.ncbi.nlm.nih.gov/pmc/articles/PMC6221888.

11 Paige Winfield Cunningham, "The Health 202: Coca-Cola Emails Reveal How Soda Industry Tries to Influence Health Officials," *Washington Post*, January 1, 2019, www.washingtonpost.com/news/powerpost/paloma/the-health-202/2019/01/29/the-health-202-coca-cola-emails-reveal-how-soda-industry-tries-to-influence-health-officials/5c4f65dd1b326b29c3778cf1; Anahad O'Connor, "Coca-Cola Funds Scientists Who Shift Blame for Obesity Away from Bad Diets," *New York Times* (Well blog), August 9, 2015, well.blogs.nytimes.com/2015/08/09/coca-cola-funds-scientists-who-shift-blame-for-obesity-away-from-bad-diets.

12 W. C. Miller, D. M. Koceja, and E. J. Hamilton, "A Meta-Analysis of the Past 25 Years of Weight Loss Research Using Diet, Exercise or Diet Plus Exercise Intervention," *International Journal of Obesity and Related Metabolic Disorders* 21, no. 10 (October 1997): 941–47, ncbi.nlm.nih.gov/pubmed/9347414.

13   "Inactivity in Obese Mice Linked to a Decreased Motivation to Move," *Science Daily*, December 29, 2016, www.sciencedaily.com/releases/2016/12/161229141901.htm.

14   "Chapter 1: Key Elements of Healthy Eating Patterns," Dietary Guidelines for Americans 2015–2020, 8th ed., Office of Disease Prevention and Health Promotion, accessed December 30, 2019, health.gov/dietaryguidelines/2015/guidelines/chapter-1/a-closer-look-inside-healthy-eating-patterns.

15   Christopher E. Ramsden et al., "Re-evaluation of the Traditional Diet-Heart Hypothesis: Analysis of Recovered Data from Minnesota Coronary Experiment (1968–73)," *BMJ* 2016 (April 12, 2016), www.bmj.com/content/353/bmj.i1246.

16   I. D. Frantz Jr. et al., "Test of Effect of Lipid Lowering by Diet on Cardiovascular Risk: The Minnesota Coronary Survey," *Arteriosclerosis* 9, no. 1 (January–February 1989): 129–35, www.ncbi.nlm.nih.gov/pubmed/2643423.

17   Anahad O'Connor, "A Decades-Old Study, Rediscovered, Challenges Advice on Saturated Fat," *New York Times,* April 13, 2016, well.blogs.nytimes.com/2016/04/13/a-decades-old-study-rediscovered-challenges-advice-on-saturated-fat.

18   Marion Nestle, "Perspective: Challenges and Controversial Issues in the Dietary Guidelines for Americans, 1980–2015." *Advances in Nutrition* 9, no. 2 (March 2018): 148–50, www.ncbi.nlm.nih.gov/pmc/articles/PMC5916425; N. Wade, "Food Board's Fat Report Hits Fire," *Science* 209, no. 4453 (July 11, 1980): 248–50, science.sciencemag.org/content/209/4453/248.

19   Gail Johnson, *Research Methods for Public Administrators*, 3rd ed. (London: Routledge, December 17, 2014).

20   Robert Klara, "Throwback Thursday: When Doctors Prescribed 'Healthy' Cigarette Brands," *Adweek*, June 18, 2015, www.adweek.com/brand-marketing/throwback-thursday-when-doctors-prescribed-healthy-cigarette-brands-165404.

21   Christopher D. Gardner et al., "Effect of Low-Fat vs Low-Carbohydrate Diet on 12-Month Weight Loss in Overweight Adults and the Association with Genotype Pattern or Insulin Secretion: The DIETFITS Randomized Clinical Trial," *JAMA* 318, no. 7 (2018) 667–79, jamanetwork.com/journals/jama/fullarticle/2673150.

22   S. J. Hur et al., "Controversy on the Correlation of Red and Processed Meat Consumption with Colorectal Cancer Risk: An Asian Perspective," *Critical Reviews in Food Science and Nutrition* 59, no. 21 (2019): 3526–37, www.ncbi.nlm.nih.gov/pubmed/29999423.

23   Rajiv Chowdhury et al., "Association of Dietary, Circulating, and Supplement Fatty Acids with Coronary Risk: A Systematic Review and Meta-analysis," *Annals of Internal Medicine* (March 18, 2014), annals.org/aim/article-abstract/1846638/association-dietary-circulating-supplement-fatty-acids-coronary-risk-systematic-review?doi=10.7326%2fM13-1788.

24   Erin E. Masterson, William R. Leonard, and Philippe P. Hujoel, "Diet, Atherosclerosis, and Helmintic Infection in Tsimane," *Lancet* 390, no. 10107 (November 4, 2017): 2034–35, www.thelancet.com/journals/lancet/article/PIIS0140-6736(17)31945-1/fulltext.

25 F. E. Morales, G. M. Tinsley, and P. M. Gordon, "Acute and Long-Term Impact of High-Protein Diets on Endocrine and Metabolic Function, Body Composition, and Exercise-Induced Adaptations," *Journal of the American College of Nutrition* 36, no. 4 (May–June 2017): 295–305, www.ncbi.nlm.nih.gov/pubmed/28443785.

26 M. S. Westerterp-Plantenga, S. G. Lemmens, and K. R. Westerterp, "Dietary Protein–Its Role in Satiety, Energetics, Weight Loss and Health," *British Journal of Nutrition* 108, no. S2 (August 2012): S105–12, www.ncbi.nlm.nih.gov/pubmed/23107521.

27 T. J. Key et al., "Dietary Habits and Mortality in 11,000 Vegetarians and Health Conscious People: Results of a 17 Year Follow Up," *BMJ* 313, no. 7060 (September 28, 1996): 775–79, www.ncbi.nlm.nih.gov/pubmed/8842068.

28 S. Mihrshahi et al., "Vegetarian Diet and All-Cause Mortality: Evidence from a Large Population-Based Australian Cohort—the 45 and Up Study," *Preventive Medicine* 97, nos. 1–7 (April 2017), www.ncbi.nlm.nih.gov/pubmed/28040519.

29 James E. Enstrom, "Health Practices and Cancer Mortality Among Active California Mormons," *Journal of the National Cancer Institute* 81 no. 23 (December 6, 1989): 1807–14, academic.oup.com/jnci/article-abstract/81/23/1807/895017; James E. Enstrom, "Cancer and Total Mortality Among Active Mormons," *Cancer* 42, no. 4 (October 1978): 1943–51, www.ncbi.nlm.nih.gov/pubmed/709540; James E. Enstrom and Lester Breslow, "Lifestyle and Reduced Mortality Among Active California Mormons, 1980–2004," *Preventive Medicine* 46, no. 2 (February 2008): 133–36, www.sciencedirect.com/science/article/pii/S0091743507003258.

30 W. H. Wilson Tang et al., "Intestinal Microbial Metabolism of Phosphatidylcholine and Cardiovascular Risk," *New England Journal of Medicine* 2013, no. 268 (2013): 1575–84, www.nejm.org/doi/10.1056/NEJMoa1109400.

31 Manuel H. Janeiro et al., "Implication of Trimethylamine N-Oxide (TMAO) in Disease: Potential Biomarker or New Therapeutic Target," *Nutrients* 10, no. 10 (October 2018): 1398, www.ncbi.nlm.nih.gov/pmc/articles/PMC6213249; Tomasz Huc et al., "Chronic, Low-Dose TMAO Treatment Reduces Diastolic Dysfunction and Heart Fibrosis in Hypertensive Rats," *American Journal of Physiology-Heart and Circulatory Physiology* (2018), doi.org/10.1152/ajpheart.00536.2018.

32 Jaime Uribarri et al., "Advanced Glycation End Products in Foods and a Practical Guide to Their Reduction in the Diet," *Journal of the American Dietary Association* 110, no. 6 (June 2010): 911–16, www.ncbi.nlm.nih.gov/pmc/articles/PMC3704564.

33 "Global Meat-Eating Is on the Rise, Bringing Surprising Benefits," *Economist*.

34 "A Century of Trends in Adult Human Height," *eLife* (July 26, 2016), https://elifesciences.org/articles/13410.

CHAPTER 5: IS MEAT A HEALTHY FOOD?

1 Fumio Watanabe et al., "Pseudovitamin B(12) Is the Predominant Cobamide of an Algal Health Food, Spirulina Tablets," *Journal of Agricultural and Food Chemistry* 47, no. 11 (November 1999): 4736–41, www.ncbi.nlm.nih.gov/pubmed/10552882.

2 Laura Tripkovic et al., "Comparison of Vitamin D$_2$ and Vitamin D$_3$ Supplementation in Raising Serum 25-Hydroxyvitamin D Status: a Systematic Review and

NOTES

Meta-analysis," *Americal Journal of Clinical Nutrition 95*, no. 6 (June 2012): 1357–64, www.ncbi.nlm.nih.gov/pmc/articles/PMC3349454.

3   "Vitamin D Fact Sheet for Health Professionals," National Institutes of Health Office of Dietary Supplements, updated August 7, 2019, ods.od.nih.gov/factsheets/VitaminD-HealthProfessional.

4   G. González-Rosendo et al., "Bioavailability of a Heme-Iron Concentrate Product Added to Chocolate Biscuit Filling in Adolescent Girls Living in a Rural Area of Mexico," *Journal of Food Science 75*, no. 3 (April 2010): H73–78, www.ncbi.nlm.nih.gov/pubmed/20492296.

5   "Classic Hereditary Hemochromatosis," Rare Disease Database, National Organization for Rare Disorders, updated 2019, rarediseases.org/rare-diseases/classic-hereditary-hemochromatosis.

6   Vazhiyil Venugopal and Kumarapanicker Gopakumar, "Shellfish: Nutritive Value, Health Benefits, and Consumer Safety," *Comprehensive Reviews in Food Science and Food Safety* (October 25, 2017), onlinelibrary.wiley.com/doi/full/10.1111/1541-4337.12312.

7   Sara M. Bronkema et al., "A Nutritional Survey of Commercially Available Grass-Finished Beef," *Meat and Muscle Biology* 2019, no. 3 (2019): 116–26, doi:10.22175/mmb2018.10.0034.

8   "Beef, Loin, Top Loin Steak, Boneless, Lip Off, Separable Lean Only, Trimmed to 0" Fat, All Grades, Raw," FoodData Central, cited October 11, 2019, fdc.nal.usda.gov/fdc-app.html#/food-details/174002/nutrients.

9   "Beef, Round, Eye of Round Roast, Boneless, Separable Lean Only, Trimmed to 0" Fat, Select, Raw," FoodData Central, cited October 11, 2019, fdc.nal.usda.gov/fdc-app.html#/food-details/334898/nutrients.

10 "Nuts, Walnuts, English," FoodData Central, cited October 11, 2019, fdc.nal.usda.gov/fdc-app.html#/food-details/170187/nutrients.

11 "Nuts, Almonds," FoodData Central, cited October 11, 2019, fdc.nal.usda.gov/fdc-app.html#/food-details/170567/nutrients.

12 "Fish, Salmon, Chinook, Raw," FoodData Central, cited October 11, 2019, fdc.nal.usda.gov/fdc-app.html#/food-details/173688/nutrients.

13 D. Średnicka-Tober et al., "Composition Differences Between Organic and Conventional Meat: A Systematic Literature Review and Meta-analysis," *British Journal of Nutrition* 2016, no. 115 (2016): 994–1011, www.ncbi.nlm.nih.gov/pubmed/26878675; H. Gerster, "Can Adults Adequately Convert Alpha-Linolenic Acid (18:3n-3) to Eicosapentaenoic Acid (20:5n-3) and Docosahexaenoic Acid 22:6n-3)?" *International Journal for Vitamin and Nutrition Research* 1998, no. 68 (1998): 159–73, www.ncbi.nlm.nih.gov/pubmed/9637947.

14 Allison J. McAfee Yeates et al., "Red Meat from Animals Offered a Grass Diet Increases Plasma and Platelet n-3 PUFA in Healthy Consumers," *British Journal of Nutrition* 105, no. 1 (January 2011): 80–89, www.researchgate.net/publication/46107212_Red_meat_from_animals_offered_a_grass_diet_increases_plasma_and_platelet_n-3_PUFA_in_healthy_consumers.

15   Bronkema et al., "A Nutritional Survey of Commercially Available Grass-Finished Beef."

16   Sarah K. Gebauer et al., "Vaccenic Acid and Trans Fatty Acid Isomers from Partially Hydrogenated Oil Both Adversely Affect LDL Cholesterol: A Double-Blind, Randomized Controlled Trial," *American Journal of Clinical Nutrition* 102, no. 6 (December 2015): 1339–46, www.ncbi.nlm.nih.gov/pubmed/26561632.

17   "Beef, Loin, Top Loin Steak," FoodData Central.

18   Centers for Disease Control and Prevention, *Surveillance for Foodborne Disease Outbreaks, United States, 2017: Annual Report* (Atlanta: US Department of Health and Human Services, 2019), www.cdc.gov/fdoss/pdf/2017_FoodBorneOutbreaks_508.pdf.

19   Narelle Fegan et al., "The Prevalence and Concentration of *Escherichia coli* O157 in Faeces of Cattle from Different Production Systems At Slaughter," *Journal of Applied Microbiol*ogy 97, no. 2 (2004): 362–70, sfamjournals.onlinelibrary.wiley.com/doi/full/10.1111/j.1365-2672.2004.02300.x.

20   Andrea Rock, "How Safe Is Your Ground Beef?" *Consumer Reports*, updated December 21, 2015, www.consumerreports.org/cro/food/how-safe-is-your-ground-beef.

21   S. Reinstein et al., "Prevalence of *Escherichia coli* O157:H7 in Organically and Naturally Raised Beef Cattle," *Applied and Environmental Microbiology* 75, no. 16 (August 2009): 5421–23, aem.asm.org/content/75/16/5421.

22   US Food & Drug Administration, "FDA Announces Implementation of GFI #213, Outlines Continuing Efforts to Address Antimicrobial Resistance," FDA.gov (since deleted, accessed via archive-it.org), January 3, 2017, wayback.archive-it.org/7993/20190423131636/https://www.fda.gov/AnimalVeterinary/NewsEvents/CVMUpdates/ucm535154.htm; Chris Dall, "FDA Reports Major Drop in Antibiotics for Food Animals," University of Minnesota Center for Infectious Disease Research and Policy, December 19, 2018, www.cidrap.umn.edu/news-perspective/2018/12/fda-reports-major-drop-antibiotics-food-animals.

23   "The Truth About: Meat and Antibiotics," Minnesota Department of Agriculture, August 19, 2019, www.health.state.mn.us/diseases/antibioticresistance/animal/truthmeat.pdf; Food Safety and Inspection Service, "United States National Residue Program for Meat, Poultry, and Egg Products FY 2018 Residue Sample Results (Red Book)," United States Department of Agriculture, www.fsis.usda.gov/wps/wcm/connect/d6baddf7-0352-4a0e-a86d-32ba2d4613ba/2018-red-book.pdf?MOD=AJPERES.

24   Tsepo Ramatla et al., "Evaluation of Antibiotic Residues in Raw Meat Using Different Analytical Methods," *Antibiotics (Basel)* 6, no. 4 (December 2017): 34, doi.org/10.3390/antibiotics6040034; H. J. Lee et al., "Prevalence of Antibiotic Residues and Antibiotic Resistance in Isolates of Chicken Meat in Korea," *Korean Journal for Food Science of Animal Resources* 38, no. 5 (October 2018): 1055–1063, doi.org/10.5851/kosfa.2018.e39.

25   Erin Jackson et al., "Adipose Tissue as a Site of Toxin Accumulation," *Comprehensive Physiology* 7, no. 4 (October 2017): 1085–135, onlinelibrary.wiley.com/doi/abs/10.1002/cphy.c160038.

26   José L. Domingo and Marti Nadal, "Carcinogenicity of Consumption of Red and Processed Meat: What About Environmental Contaminants?" *Environmental Research* 145 (February 2016): 109–15, www.ncbi.nlm.nih.gov/pubmed/26656511; José L Domingo, "Concentrations of Environmental Organic Contaminants in Meat and Meat Products and Human Dietary Exposure: A Review," *Food and Chemical Toxicology* 107, part A (September 2017): 20–26, www.sciencedirect.com/science/article/pii/S027869151730340X.

27   Alison L. Van Eenennaam and A. E. Young, "Detection of Dietary DNA, Protein, and Glyphosate in Meat, Milk, and Eggs," *Journal of Animal Science* 95, no. 7 (July 2017): 3247–69, academic.oup.com/jas/article/95/7/3247/4702986.

28   Karina Schnabel et al., "Effects of Glyphosate Residues and Different Concentrate Feed Proportions on Performance, Energy Metabolism and Health Characteristics in Lactating Dairy Cows," *Archives of Animal Nutrition* 71, no. 6 (2017): 413–427, www.tandfonline.com/doi/abs/10.1080/1745039X.2017.1391487?journalCode=gaan20.

29   Temple Grandin, "The Effect of Stress on Livestock and Meat Quality Prior to and During Slaughter," *International Journal for the Study of Animal Problems* 1, no. 5 (1980): 313–37, animalstudiesrepository.org/acwp_faafp/20/.

30   "U.S. Food-Away-from-Home Spending Continued to Outpace Food-at-Home Spending in 2018," United States Department of Agriculture, updated August 26, 2019, www.ers.usda.gov/data-products/chart-gallery/gallery/chart-detail/?chartId=58364.

31   Eddie Yoon, "The Grocery Industry Confronts a New Problem: Only 10% of Americans Love Cooking," *Harvard Business Review*, September 22, 2017, hbr.org/2017/09/the-grocery-industry-confronts-a-new-problem-only-10-of-americans-love-cooking.

32   Alex Morrell and Skye Gould, "A Close Look at Americans' Food Budget Shows an Obvious Place to Save Money," Business Insider, February 17, 2017, www.businessinsider.com/americans-spending-food-bls-2017-2.

33   Sarah Treuhaft and Allison Karpyn, "The Grocery Gap: Who Has Access to Healthy Food and Why It Matters," The Food Trust, 2010, accessed December 31, 2019, thefoodtrust.org/uploads/media_items/grocerygap.original.pdf.

CHAPTER 6: EVEN IF MEAT ISN'T BAD FOR ME, CAN'T I GET ALL MY NUTRITION FROM PLANTS?

1   Jay R. Hoffman and Michael J. Falvo, "Protein—Which Is Best?" *Journal of Sports Science & Medicine* 3, no. 3 (September 2004): 118–30, www.ncbi.nlm.nih.gov/pmc/articles/PMC3905294/table/table001/.

2   Ghulam Sarwar, "The Protein Digestibility-Corrected Amino Acid Score Method Overestimates Quality of Proteins Containing Antinutritional Factors and of Poorly Digestible Proteins Supplemented with Limiting Amino Acids in Rats," *Journal of Nutrition* 127, no. 5 (May 1997): 758–64, www.ncbi.nlm.nih.gov/pubmed/9164998.

NOTES

3   Martial Dangin et al., "The Rate of Protein Digestion Affects Protein Gain Differently During Aging in Humans," *Journal of Physiology* 549, no. 2 (2003): 635–44, www.eatrightnc.org/assets/webinar-january-spano/the%20rate%20of%20protein%20digestion%20affects%20protein%20gain%20differently%20in%20aged%20humans.pdf; David C. Dallas et al., "Personalizing Protein Nourishment," *Critical Reviews in Food Science and Nourishment* 57, no. 15 (2017): 3313–31, www.ncbi.nlm.nih.gov/pmc/articles/PMC4927412/.

4   Hoffman and Falvo, "Protein—Which Is Best?," 118–30.

5   Tanya L. Blasbalg et al., "Changes in Consumption of Omega-3 and Omega-6 Fatty Acids in the United States During the 20th Century," *American Journal of Clinical Nutrition* 93, no. 5 (May 2011): 950–62, academic.oup.com/ajcn/article/93/5/950/4597940/.

6   Hannah E. Theobald, "Dietary Calcium and Health," *Nutrition Bulletin* 30, no. 3 (September 2005): 237–77, onlinelibrary.wiley.com/doi/10.1111/j.1467-3010.2005.00514.x/full#b62.

7   Adrian R. West and Phillip S. Oates, "Mechanisms of Heme Iron Absorption: Current Questions and Controversies," *World Journal of Gastroenterology* 14, no. 26 (July 2008): 4101–10, www.ncbi.nlm.nih.gov/pmc/articles/PMC2725368/.

8   Handan Akçakaya et al., "β-carotene Treatment Alters the Cellular Death Process in Oxidative Stress-Induced K562 Cells," *Cell Biology International* 41, no. 3 (March 2017): 309–19, www.ncbi.nlm.nih.gov/pubmed/28035721; Sharada H. Sharma, Senthilkumar Thulasingam, and Sangeetha Nagarajan, "Terpenoids as Anti-colon Cancer Agents—A Comprehensive Review on Its Mechanistic Perspectives," *European Journal of Pharmacology* 795 (January 25, 2017): 169–78, www.ncbi.nlm.nih.gov/pubmed/27940056.

9   Monica H. Carlsen et al., "The Total Antioxidant Content of More Than 3100 Foods, Beverages, Spices, Herbs and Supplements Used Worldwide," *Nutrition Journal* 9, no. 3 (2010), www.ncbi.nlm.nih.gov/pmc/articles/PMC2841576/.

10   Goran Bjelakovic et al., "Antioxidant Supplements for Prevention of Gastrointestinal Cancers: A Systematic Review and Meta-analysis," *Lancet* 364, no. 9441 (October 2004): 1219–28, www.ncbi.nlm.nih.gov/pubmed/15464182.

11   Michelle Yu, "Most Vitamins Are from China—It's a Bigger Problem Than You Realize," Epoch Times, February 6, 2014, www.theepochtimes.com/5-facts-you-need-to-know-if-your-vitamins-are-from-china_361599.html.

12   Lilian U. Thompson, "Potential Health Benefits and Problems Associated with Antinutrients in Foods," *Food Research International* 26, no. 2 (1993): 131–49, www.sciencedirect.com/science/article/pii/096399699390069U.

13   H. Walter Lopez et al., "Minerals and Phytic Acid Interactions: Is It a Real Problem for Human Nutrition?" *International Journal of Food Science and Technology* (September 2002), onlinelibrary.wiley.com/doi/10.1046/j.1365-2621.2002.00618.x/full.

14   Nevin S. Scrimshaw, "Iron Deficiency," *Scientific American* 265, no. 4 (October 1991): 46–52, www.ncbi.nlm.nih.gov/pubmed/1745900.

NOTES

15   Ludmila Křížová et al., "Isoflavones," *Molecules* 24, no. 6 (March 2019): 1076, doi.org/10.3390/molecules24061076; Xiao-xue Yuan et al., "Effects of Soybean Isoflavones on Reproductive Parameters in Chinese Mini-Pig Boars," *Journal of Animal Science and Biotechnology* 3, no. 1 (2012): 31, doi.org/10.1186/2049-1891-3-31.

16   Christopher R. Cederroth et al., "Soy, Phyto-oestrogens and Male Reproductive Function: A Review," *International Journal of Andrology* 33, no. 2 (April 2010): 304–16, onlinelibrary.wiley.com/doi/10.1111/j.1365-2605.2009.01011.x/full.

17   X Gu et al., "Identification of IgE-Binding Proteins in Soy Lecithin," *International Archives of Allergy and Immunology* 126, no. 3 (2001), www.karger.com/Article/Abstract/49517.

18   Joanne M. Bell and Paula K. Lundberg, "Effects of a Commercial Soy Lecithin Preparation on Development of Sensorimotor Behavior and Brain Biochemistry in the Rat," *Developmental Psychobiology* 18, no. 1 (January 1985): 59–66, www.ncbi.nlm.nih.gov/pubmed/4038491.

19   G. Padama and Keith H. Steinkraus, "Cyanide Detoxification in Cassava for Food and Feed Uses," *Critical Reviews in Food Science and Nutrition* 35, no. 4 (July 1995): 299–339, www.ncbi.nlm.nih.gov/pubmed/7576161.

20   Robin R. White and Mary Beth Hall, "Nutritional and Greenhouse Gas Impacts of Removing Animals from US Agriculture," *PNAS* 114, no. 48 (November 28, 2017), www.pnas.org/content/114/48/E10301.

21   W. C. Leung et al., "Two Common Single Nucleotide Polymorphisms in the Gene Encoding β-Carotene 15,15'-Monoxygenase Alter β-Carotene Metabolism in Female Volunteers," *FASEB Journal* 23, no. 4 (April 2009): 1041–53, www.ncbi.nlm.nih.gov/pubmed/19103647; Guangwen Tang, "Bioconversion of Dietary Provitamin A Carotenoids to Vitamin A in Humans," *American Journal of Clinical Nutrition* 91, no. 5 (May 2010): 1468S–1473S, www.ncbi.nlm.nih.gov/pmc/articles/PMC2854912/.

22   Abir Zakaria, Inas Sabry, and Amal El Shehaby, "Glycemic Control in Insulin Treated Type 2 Diabetes Mellitus Patients: Ramadan-like Fasting Reduces Carbonyl Stress and Improves Glycemic Control in Insulin Treated Type 2 Diabetes Mellitus Patients," *Life Science Journal* 10, no. 384 (January 2013), www.researchgate.net/publication/261879563_Ramadan-Like_Fasting_Reduces_Carbonyl_Stress_and_Improves_Glycemic_Control_in_Insulin_Treated_Type_2_Diabetes_Mellitus_Patients; Michelle N. Harvie et al., "The Effects of Intermittent or Continuous Energy Restriction on Weight Loss and Metabolic Disease Risk Markers: A Randomized Trial in Young Overweight Women," *International Journal of Obesity* 35, no. 5 (May 2011): 714–27, www.ncbi.nlm.nih.gov/pubmed/20921964.

23   A. M. J. Gilsing et al., "Serum Concentrations of Vitamin B12 and Folate in British Male Omnivores, Vegetarians and Vegans: Results from a Cross-Sectional Analysis of the EPIC-Oxford Cohort Study," *European Journal of Clinical Nutrition* 64, no. 9 (September 2010): 933–39, www.ncbi.nlm.nih.gov/pubmed/20648045.

24   Wolfgang Herrmann, "Vitamin B 12 Deficiency in Vegetarians," *Vegetarian and Plant-Based Diets in Health and Disease Prevention* (December 2017), www.researchgate.net/publication/317337523_Vitamin_B_12_Deficiency_in_Vegetarians.

25 Christian Lachner, Nanette I. Steinle, and William T. Regenold, "The Neuropsychiatry of Vitamin B12 Deficiency in Elderly Patients," *Journal of Neuropsychiatry and Clinical Neurosciences* 24, no. 1 (Winter 2012): 5–15, www.ncbi.nlm.nih.gov/pubmed/22450609.

26 Watanabe et al., "Pseudovitamin B12," 4736–41.

27 "Global Anaemia Prevalence and Number of Individuals Affected," World Health Organization, accessed December 30, 2019, www.who.int/vmnis/anaemia/prevalence/summary/anaemia_data_status_t2/en/.

28 Lisa M. Haider et al., "The Effect of Vegetarian Diets on Iron Status in Adults: A Systematic Review and Meta-analysis," *Critical Reviews in Food Science and Nutrition* 58, no. 8 (May 24, 2018): 1359–74, www.ncbi.nlm.nih.gov/pubmed/27880062.

29 Ruby Nyika, "More Spent on Low Iron Hospitalisations as Meat Intake Declines," Stuff, January 1, 2019, www.stuff.co.nz/national/health/108767316/more-spent-on-low-iron-hospitalisations-as-meat-intake-declines.

30 Scrimshaw, "Iron Deficiency," 46–52.

31 Tue H. Hansen at al., "Bone Turnover, Calcium Homeostasis, and Vitamin D Status in Danish Vegans," *European Journal of Clinical Nutrition* 72, no. 7 (July 2018): 1046–54, www.ncbi.nlm.nih.gov/pubmed/29362456.

32 Winston John Craig, "Nutrition Concerns and Health Effects of Vegetarian Diets," *Nutrition in Clinical Practice* 25, no. 6 (December 2010): 613–20, www.ncbi.nlm.nih.gov/pubmed/21139125.

33 Connie M. Weaver, William R. Proulx, and Robert Heaney, "Choices for Achieving Adequate Dietary Calcium with a Vegetarian Diet," *American Journal of Clinical Nutrition* 70, no. 3 (September 1999), academic.oup.com/ajcn/article/70/3/543s/4714998.

34 Anna-Liisa Elorinne et al., "Food and Nutrient Intake and Nutritional Status of Finnish Vegans and Non-vegetarians," *PLOS One* 11, no. 3 (February 3, 2016), journals.plos.org/plosone/article?id=10.1371/journal.pone.0148235.

35 Isabel Iguacel et al., "Veganism, Vegetarianism, Bone Mineral Density, and Fracture Risk: A Systematic Review and Meta-analysis," *Nutrition Reviews* 77, no. 1 (January 2019): 1–18, www.ncbi.nlm.nih.gov/pubmed/30376075; Paul N. Appleby et al., "Comparative Fracture Risk in Vegetarians and Nonvegetarians in EPIC-Oxford," *European Journal of Clinical Nutrition* 61 (2007): 1400–6, www.nature.com/articles/1602659.

36 Anne Lise Brantsæter et al., "Inadequate Iodine Intake in Population Groups Defined by Age, Life Stage and Vegetarian Dietary Practice in a Norwegian Convenience Sample," *Nutrients* 10, no. 2 (February 17, 2018): E230, www.ncbi.nlm.nih.gov/pubmed/29462974.

37 Umesh Kapil, "Health Consequences of Iodine Deficiency," *Sultan Qaboos University Medical Journal* 7, no. 3 (December 2007): 267–72, www.ncbi.nlm.nih.gov/pmc/articles/PMC3074887/.

38 Zahra Solati et al., "Zinc Monotherapy Increases Serum Brain-Derived Neurotrophic Factor (BDNF) Levels and Decreases Depressive Symptoms in Overweight

or Obese Subjects: A Double-Blind, Randomized, Placebo-Controlled Trial," *Nutritional Neuroscience* 18, no. 4 (May 2015): 162–68, www.ncbi.nlm.nih.gov/pubmed/24621065.

39 Erik Messamore and Robert K. McNamara, "Detection and Treatment of Omega-3 Fatty Acid Deficiency in Psychiatric Practice: Rationale and Implementation," *Lipids in Health and Disease* 15 (2016), lipidworld.biomedcentral.com/articles/10.1186/s12944-016-0196-5.

40 Presentation by Georgia Ede; Zahra Solati et al., "Zinc Monotherapy"; Darryl W. Eyles, Thomas H. J. Burne, and John J. McGrath, "Vitamin D, Effects on Brain Development, Adult Brain Function and the Links Between Low Levels of Vitamin D and Neuropsychiatric Disease," *Frontiers in Neuroendocrinology* 34, no. 1 (2013): 47–64, doi.org/10.1016/j.yfrne.2012.07.001; Lachner et al., "The Neuropsychiatry of Vitamin B12 Deficiency in Elderly Patients," 5–15; Jonghan Kim and Marianne Wessling-Resnick, "Iron and Mechanisms of Emotional Behavior," *Journal of Nutritional Biochemistry* 25, no. 11 (2014): 1101–7, doi.org/10.1016/j.jnutbio.2014.07.003; Shaheen E. Lakhan and Karen F. Vieira, "Nutritional Therapies for Mental Disorders," *Nutrition Journal* 7, no. 2 (2008), doi.org/10.1186/1475-2891-7-2.

41 Caroline Rae et al., "Oral Creatine Monohydrate Supplementation Improves Brain Performance: A Double-Blind, Placebo-Controlled, Cross-Over Trial," *Proceedings of the Royal Society B* 270, no. 1529 (October 22, 2003), royalsocietypublishing.org/doi/abs/10.1098/rspb.2003.2492.

42 T. A. B. Sanders and Sheela Reddy, "The Influence of a Vegetarian Diet on the Fatty Acid Composition of Human Milk and the Essential Fatty Acid Status of the Infant," *Journal of Pediatrics* 120, no. 4, part 2 (April 1992): S71–77, www.jpeds.com/article/S0022-3476(05)81239-9/pdf.

43 Sheela Reddy, T. A. B. Sanders, and O. Obeid, "The Influence of Maternal Vegetarian Diet on Essential Fatty Acid Status of the Newborn," *European Journal of Clinical Nutrition* 48, no. 5 (May 1004): 358–68, www.ncbi.nlm.nih.gov/pubmed/8055852.

44 Robert J. Williams and Susan P. Gloster, "Human Sex Ratio as It Relates to Caloric Availability," *Biodemography and Social Biology* 39, nos. 3–4 (1992): 285–91, www.tandfonline.com/doi/abs/10.1080/19485565.1992.9988823.

45 P. Hudson and R. Buckley, "Vegetarian Diets: Are They Good for Pregnant Women and Their Babies?," *Practising Midwife* 3, no. 7 (June 30, 2000): 22–23, europepmc.org/abstract/med/12026434.

46 Nathan Cofnas, "Is Vegetarianism Healthy for Children?," *Critical Reviews in Food Science and Nutrition* 59, no. 13 (2019): 2052–60, www.tandfonline.com/doi/full/10.1080/10408398.2018.1437024?src=recsys.

47 "Avis de l'ARMB sur le véganisme des enfants," Union professionnelle des diététiciens de langue française, May 16, 2019, updlf-asbl.be/articles/avis-de-larmb-sur-le-veganisme-des-enfants.

48 "Vegan Couple Sentenced to Life over Baby's Death," NBC News, May 9, 2007, www.nbcnews.com/id/18574603/ns/us_news-crime_and_courts/t/vegan-couple-sentenced-life-over-babys-death.

49 "Baby Death: Parents Convicted over Vegetable Milk Diet," BBC News, June 14, 2017, www.bbc.com/news/world-europe-40274493.

50 Mary Hui, "An Italian Baby Raised on a Vegan Diet Is Hospitalized for Malnutrition," *Washington Post*, July 11, 2016, www.washingtonpost.com/news/morning-mix/wp/2016/07/11/italian-baby-fed-vegan-diet-hospitalized-for-malnutrition/.

51 C. Roed, F. Skovby, and A. M. Lund, "Severe Vitamin B12 Deficiency in Infants Breastfed by Vegans" [in Danish], *Ugeskrift for Laeger* 171, no. 43 (October 19, 2009): 3099–101, www.ncbi.nlm.nih.gov/pubmed/19852900.

52 A. Mariani et al., "Conséquences de l'allaitement maternel exclusif chez le nouveau-né de mère végétalienne—À propos d'un cas" [Consequences of exclusive breast-feeding in vegan mother newborn—Case report], *Archives de Pédiatrie* 16, no. 11 (November 2009): 1461–63, www.ncbi.nlm.nih.gov/pubmed/19748244.

53 Paulina J. Bravo, Judith C. Ibarra, and Marcela M. Paredes, "Hematological and Neurological Compromise Due to Vitamin B12 Deficit in Infant of a Vegetarian Mother: Case Report" [in Spanish], *Revista Chilena de Pediatria* 85, no. 3 (May 31, 2014): 337–43, europepmc.org/abstract/med/25697251.

54 A. M. Lund, "Questions About a Vegan Diet Should Be Included in Differential Diagnostics of Neurologically Abnormal Infants with Failure to Thrive," *Acta Pædiatrica* (April 21, 2019), onlinelibrary.wiley.com/doi/abs/10.1111/apa.14805.

55 Judie L. Hulett et al., "Animal Source Foods Have a Positive Impact on the Primary School Test Scores of Kenyan Schoolchildren in a Cluster-Randomised, Controlled Feeding Intervention Trial," *British Journal of Nutrition* 111, no. 5 (March 14, 2014): 875–86, doi.org/10.1017/S0007114513003310.

56 L. M. Petit, A. Nydeggar, and P. Müller, "Vegan Diet in Children: What Potential Deficits to Monitor?" [in French], *Revue Medicale Suisse* 15, no. 638 (February 13, 2019): 373–75, www.ncbi.nlm.nih.gov/pubmed/30762997.

CHAPTER 8: CAN A SUSTAINABLE FOOD SYSTEM EXIST WITHOUT ANIMALS?

1 Carolyn S. Mattick et al., "Anticipatory Life Cycle Analysis of *In Vitro* Biomass Cultivation for Cultured Meat Production in the United States," *Environmental Science & Technology* 49, no. 19 (October 6, 2015): 11941–49, pubs.acs.org/doi/10.1021/acs.est.5b01614.

CHAPTER 9: ARE CATTLE CONTRIBUTING TO CLIMATE CHANGE?

1 "Understanding Global Warming Potentials," Greenhouse Gas Emissions, United States Environmental Protection Agency, accessed December 31, 2019, www.epa.gov/ghgemissions/understanding-global-warming-potentials.

NOTES

2   Irene Piccini et al., "Greenhouse Gas Emissions from Dung Pats Vary with Dung Beetle Species and with Assemblage Composition," *PLOS One* (July 12, 2017), journals.plos. org/plosone/article?id=10.1371/journal.pone.0178077; Eleanor M. Slade et al., "The Role of Dung Beetles in Reducing Greenhouse Gas Emissions from Cattle Farming," *Scientific Reports* 6 (2016), www.nature.com/articles/srep18140.

3   "Time Line of the American Bison," United States Fish and Wildlife Service, accessed December 31, 2019, www.fws.gov/bisonrange/timeline.htm; Alexander N. Hristov, "Historic, Pre-European Settlement, and Present-Day Contribution of Wild Ruminants to Enteric Methane Emissions in the United States," *Journal of Animal Science* 90, no. 4 (April 2012): 1371–75, www.ncbi.nlm.nih.gov/pubmed/22178852; "Elk Facts," Rocky Mountain Elk Foundation Elk Network, accessed December 31, 2019, elknetwork.com/elkfacts/; David Petersen, "North American Deer: Mule, Whitetail and Coastal Blacktail Deer," *Mother Earth News,* November/December 1985, www. motherearthnews.com/nature-and-environment/north-american-deer-zmaz85ndzgoe; G. A. Feldhamer, B. C. Thompson, and J. A. Chapman, eds., *Wild Mammals of North America* (Baltimore: Johns Hopkins University Press, 2003); IUCN SSC Antelope Specialist Group 2016, "Pronghorn (Antilocapra americana)," *The IUCN Red List of Threatened Species,* June 14, 2016, dx.doi.org/10.2305/IUCN.UK.2016-3.RLTS. T1677A50181848.en.

4   Hristov, "Historic, Pre-European Settlement," 1371–75.

5   "Belching Ruminants, a Minor Player in Atmospheric Methane," Joint FAO/IAEA Programme, accessed December 31, 2019, www-naweb.iaea.org/nafa/aph/stories/2008-atmospheric-methane.html.

6   Carol Rasmussen, "NASA-Led Study Solves a Methane Puzzle," NASA, January 2, 2018, www.nasa.gov/feature/jpl/nasa-led-study-solves-a-methane-puzzle/.

7   Heinz-Ulrich Neue, "Methane Emission from Rice Fields: Wetland Rice Fields May Make a Major Contribution to Global Warming," *BioScience* 43, no. 7 (1993): 466–73, www.ciesin.org/docs/004-032/004-032.html.

8   Kritee Kritee et al., "High Nitrous Oxide Fluxes from Rice Indicate the Need to Manage Water for Both Long- and Short-Term Climate Impacts," *PNAS* 115, no. 39 (September 25, 2018): 9720–25, www.pnas.org/content/115/39/9720.

9   Cardiff University, "Baltic Clams and Worms Release as Much Greenhouse Gas as 20,000 Dairy Cows," Phys.org, October 13, 2017, phys.org/news/2017-10-baltic-clams-worms-greenhouse-gas.html; emphasis added.

10 Jenny Stiernstedt, "MP Proposal: Shoot More Moose—for the Sake of Climate" [in Swedish], Svenska Dagbladet, May 22, 2017, www.svd.se/mp-forslag-skjut-fler-algar --for-klimatets-skull/om/mp-kongressen-2017.

11 C. Alan Rotz et al., "Environmental Footprints of Beef Cattle Production in the United States," *Agricultural Systems* 169 (February 2019): 1–13, www.sciencedirect.com/ science/article/pii/S0308521X18305675.

12 R. Goodland and J. Anhang, "Livestock and Climate Change: What If the Key Actors in Climate Change Are . . . Cows, Pigs, and Chickens?," *Worldwatch* 22, no. 6 (2009): 11, www.cabdirect.org/cabdirect/abstract/20093312389.

13 Frank Mitloehner, "Livestock and Climate Change," UC Davis College of Agricultural and Environmental Sciences, April 29, 2016, caes.ucdavis.edu/news/articles/2016/04/livestock-and-climate-change-facts-and-fiction.

14 Xiaochi Zhou et al., "Estimation of Methane Emissions from the U.S. Ammonia Fertilizer Industry Using a Mobile Sensing Approach," *Elementa: Science of the Anthropocene* 7, no. 1 (May 28, 2019), www.elementascience.org/articles/10.1525/elementa.358/.

15 W. R. Teague et al., "The Role of Ruminants in Reducing Agriculture's Carbon Footprint in North America," *Journal of Soil and Water Conservation* 71, no. 2 (March/April 2016): 156–64, www.jswconline.org/content/71/2/156.full.pdf+html.

16 William J. Parton et al., "Measuring and Mitigating Agricultural Greenhouse Gas Production in the US Great Plains, 1870–2000," *PNAS* 112, no. 34 (August 25, 2015), www.pnas.org/content/112/34/E4681.

17 Todd A. Ontl and Lisa A. Schulte, "Soil Carbon Storage," *Nature Education Knowledge* 3, no. 10 (2012): 35, www.nature.com/scitable/knowledge/library/soil-carbon-storage-84223790.

18 Eelco Rohling, "We Need to Get Rid of Carbon in the Atmosphere, Not Just Reduce Emissions," The Conversation, April 19, 2017, theconversation.com/we-need-to-get-rid-of-carbon-in-the-atmosphere-not-just-reduce-emissions-72573.

19 Paige L. Stanley et al., "Impacts of Soil Carbon Sequestration on Life Cycle Greenhouse Gas Emissions in Midwestern USA Beef Finishing Systems," *Agricultural Systems* 162 (May 2018): 249–58, www.sciencedirect.com/science/article/pii/S0308521X17310338

20 J. E. Rowntree et al., "Ecosystem Impacts and Productive Capacity of a Multispecies Pastured Livestock System," *Frontiers in Sustainable Food Systems* (in review, 2020).

21 E. F. Viglizzo et al., "Reassessing the Role of Grazing Lands in Carbon-Balance Estimations: Meta-analysis and Review," *Science of the Total Environment* 661 (April 15, 2019): 531–42, www.sciencedirect.com/science/article/pii/S0048969719301470.

22 White and Hall, "Nutritional and Greenhouse Gas Impacts of Removing Animals from US Agriculture."

23 Ryan Reuter, Matt Beck, and Logan Thompson, "What Are Enteric Methane Emissions?," Beefresearch.org, 2017, www.beefresearch.org/CMDocs/BeefResearch/Sustainability_FactSheet_TopicBriefs/ToughQA/FS17Methane.pdf.

CHAPTER 10: AREN'T CATTLE INEFFICIENT WITH FEED?

1 Jeanne Yacoubou, "Factors Involved in Calculating Grain: Meat Conversion Ratios," Vegetarian Resource Group, accessed December 31, 2019, www.vrg.org/environment/grain_meat_conversion_ratios.php.

2 Rotz et al., "Environmental Footprints of Beef Cattle," 1–13.

3 National Academies of Sciences, Engineering, and Medicine, *Nutrient Requirements of Beef Cattle*, 8th rev. ed. (Washington, DC: National Academies Press, 2016), www.nap.edu/catalog/19014/nutrient-requirements-of-beef-cattle-eighth-revised-edition.

4   Anne Mottet et al., "Livestock: On Our Plates or Eating at Our Table? A New Analysis of the Feed/Food Debate," *Global Food Security* 14 (January 2017), www.researchgate.net/publication/312201313_Livestock_On_our_plates_or_eating_at_our_table_A_new_analysis_of_the_feedfood_debate.

5   Daniel L. Marti, Rachel J. Johnson, and Kenneth H. Mathews, Jr., "Where's the (Not) Meat?: Byproducts from Beef and Pork Production," United States Department of Agriculture Economic Research Service, accessed December 31, 2019, www.ers.usda.gov/webdocs/publications/37427/8801_ldpm20901.pdf?v=0.

6   Daniel Gade, "II.G.13—Hogs (Pigs)," in *The Cambridge World History of Food*, vol. 1, ed. Kenneth F. Kiple (New York: Cambridge University Press, 2000), 537.

7   Gade, "II.G.13—Hogs (Pigs)," 538.

8   "The Pig Idea," Feedback Global, accessed December 31, 2019, feedbackglobal.org/campaigns/pig-idea/.

9   "Key Facts on Food Loss and Waste You Should Know!" SAVE FOOD: Global Initiative on Food Loss and Waste Reduction, Food and Agriculture Organization of the United Nations, accessed December 31, 2019, www.fao.org/save-food/resources/keyfindings/en/.

10   "Pig Idea," Feedback Global.

CHAPTER 11: DON'T CATTLE TAKE UP TOO MUCH LAND?

1   "Crop Production and Natural Resource Use," in *World Agriculture: Towards 2015/2030, An FAO Perspective* (FAO, 2003), www.fao.org/3/y4252e/y4252e06.htm.

2   Jeffrey Sayer and Kenneth G. Cassman, "Agricultural Innovation to Protect the Environment," *PNAS* 110, no. 21 (May 21, 2013), www.pnas.org/content/110/21/8345.

3   Dan Charles, "Iowa Farmers Look to Trap Carbon in Soil," NPR, July 15, 2007, www.npr.org/templates/story/story.php?storyId=11951725.

4   Gil Gullickson, "Indigo AG Announces the Terraton Initiative That Pays Farmers for Carbon Sequestration," Successful Farming, June 12, 2019, www.agriculture.com/news/crops/indigo-ag-announces-the-terraton-initiative-that-pays-farmers-for-carbon-sequestration.

5   "Livestock on Grazing Lands" in *Livestock & the Environment: Meeting the Challenge* (FAO), accessed December 31, 2019, www.fao.org/3/x5304e/x5304e03.htm.

6   "Crop Production and Natural Resource Use."

7   H. Eswaran, R. Lal, and P. F. Reich, "Land Degradation: An Overview," in *Responses to Land Degradation*, ed. EM Bridges et al., (New Delhi: Oxford Press, 2001), www.nrcs.usda.gov/wps/portal/nrcs/detail/soils/use/?cid=nrcs142p2_054028.

8   "Crop Production and Natural Resource Use."

9   "DROUGHT: Monitoring Economic, Environmental, and Social Impacts," National Centers for Environmental Information, accessed December 31, 2019, www.ncdc.noaa.gov/news/drought-monitoring-economic-environmental-and-social-impacts; USGCRP,

"Precipitation Change in the United States," in *Climate Change Special Report: Fourth National Climate Assessment*, vol. 1, ed. D. J. Wuebbles et al. (Washington, DC: US Global Change Research Program, 2017), science2017.globalchange.gov/chapter/7/.

10 Mottet et al., "Livestock."

11 Mottet et al.

12 Richard Florida, "Why Bigger Cities Are Greener," Citylab.com, April 19, 2012, www.citylab.com/life/2012/04/why-bigger-cities-are-greener/863/.

13 Christopher Bren d'Amour et al., "Future Urban Land Expansion and Implications for Global Croplands," *PNAS* 114, no. 34 (August 22, 2017): 8939–44, www.pnas.org/content/114/34/8939.

14 "U.S. Bioenergy Statistics," United States Department of Agriculture Economic Research Service, December 6, 2019, www.ers.usda.gov/data-products/us-bioenergy-statistics/.

15 Chris Arsenault, "Only 60 Years of Farming Left If Soil Degradation Continues," *Scientific American*, December 5, 2014, www.scientificamerican.com/article/only-60-years-of-farming-left-if-soil-degradation-continues/

16 Eswaran, Lal, and Reich, "Land Degradation."

17 Eswaran, Lal, and Reich.

18 P. J. Gerber et al., *Tackling Climate Change Through Livestock—A Global Assessment of Emissions and Mitigation Opportunities* (Rome: Food and Agriculture Organization of the United Nations, 2003), www.fao.org/3/a-i3437e.pdf.

CHAPTER 12: DON'T CATTLE DRINK TOO MUCH WATER?

1 Arjen Y. Hoekstra et al., "Grey Water Footprint," in *The Water Footprint Assessment Manual: Setting the Global Standard* (London: Earthscan, 2011), waterfootprint.org/en/water-footprint/glossary/#GrWF.

2 Mesfin M. Mekonnen and Arjen Y. Hoekstra, "The Green, Blue, and Grey Water Footprint of Farm Animals and Animal Products," Value of Water Research Report Series 48, UNESCO-IHE (2010), waterfootprint.org/media/downloads/Report-48-WaterFootprint-AnimalProducts-Vol1.pdf.

3 Jude Capper, "Is the Grass Always Greener? Comparing Resource Use and Carbon Footprints of Conventional, Natural and Grass-Fed Beef Production Systems," *Animals* 2 (2012): 127–43, www.researchgate.net/publication/274614830_Is_the_grass_always_greener_Comparing_resource_use_and_carbon_footprints_of_conventional_natural_and_grass-fed_beef_production_systems.

4 Rotz et al., "Environmental Footprints of Beef Cattle," 1–13.

5 "2012 Quivira Coalition Conference, Sandra Postel—Water," posted by Quivira Coalition, YouTube, December 17, 2012, www.youtube.com/watch?v=agSMj2KC708.

6 Michel Doreau, Michael S. Corson, and Stephen G. Wiedemann, "Water Use by Livestock: A Global Perspective for a Regional Issue?," *Animal Frontiers* 2, no. 2 (April 2012): 9–16, academic.oup.com/af/article/2/2/9/4638620.

NOTES

7   Ashley Brooks et al., "Does Beef Really Use That Much Water?," Beefresearch.org, 2015, www.beefresearch.org/CMDocs/BeefResearch/Sustainability_FactSheet_TopicBriefs/ToughQA/FS2Water.pdf.

8   Dave Berndtson, "As Global Groundwater Disappears, Rice, Wheat and Other International Crops May Start to Vanish," *PBS News Hour*, April 17, 2017. https://www.pbs.org/newshour/science/global-groundwater-disappears-rice-wheat-international-crops-may-start-vanish.

9   Mesfin M. Mekonnen and Arjen Y. Hoekstra, "A Global Assessment of the Water Foot print of Farm Animal Products," *Ecosystems* 15 (2012): 405–15, waterfootprint.org/media/downloads/Mekonnen-Hoekstra-2012-WaterFootprintFarmAnimalProducts.pdf.

10   "Irrigation Water Use," US Geological Survey, USGS.gov, accessed December 31, 2019, www.usgs.gov/special-topic/water-science-school/science/irrigation-water-use.

11   "Irrigation Water Use."

12   James S. Famiglietti, "The Global Groundwater Crisis," *Nature Climate Change* 4 (2014): 945–48, www.nature.com/articles/nclimate2425.

13   Food and Drug Administration, "2011 Report on Antimicrobials Sold or Distributed for Use in Food-Producing Animals," September 2014, www.fda.gov/downloads/ForIndustry/UserFees/AnimalDrugUserFeeActADUFA/UCM338170.pdf.

14   Michael J. Martin, Sapna E. Thottathil, and Thomas B. Newman, "Antibiotics Overuse in Animal Agriculture: A Call to Action for Health Care Providers," *American Journal of Public Health* 105, no. 12 (December 2015): 2409–10, www.ncbi.nlm.nih.gov/pmc/articles/PMC4638249/.

15   Bonnie M. Marshall and Stuart B. Levy, "Food Animals and Antimicrobials: Impacts on Human Health," *Clinical Microbiology Reviews* 24, no. 4 (October 2011): 718–33, www.ncbi.nlm.nih.gov/pmc/articles/PMC3194830/.

CHAPTER 13: IS EATING ANIMALS IMMORAL?

1   Chris Ip, "Impossible Foods' Rising Empire of Almost-Meat," *Engadget*, May 19, 2019, www.engadget.com/2019/05/19/impossible-foods-burger-sausage-empire.

2   Maggie Germano, "Despite Their Priorities, Nearly Half of Americans Over 55 Still Don't Have a Will," *Forbes*, February 15, 2019, www.forbes.com/sites/maggiegermano/2019/02/15/despite-their-priorities-nearly-half-of-americans-over-55-still-dont-have-a-will/#3573b5585238.

3   Wesley J. Smith, "Here's a Dumb Idea: To Eliminate All Suffering, Eliminate Predators!," Evolution News, July 31, 2014, evolutionnews.org/2014/07/heres_a_dumb_id/.

4   Natalie Wolchover, Quanta Magazine, "A New Physics Theory of Life," *Scientific American*, January 28, 2014, www.scientificamerican.com/article/a-new-physics-theory-of-life/.

5   Dan Bilefsky, "Inky the Octopus Escapes from a New Zealand Aquarium," *New York Times*, April 13, 2016, www.nytimes.com/2016/04/14/world/asia/inky-octopus-new-zealand-aquarium.html.

6   "Octopus Takes Pictures of Visitors at New Zealand Aquarium," YouTube, April 13, 2015. www.youtube.com/watch?v=_Cs5rJidznQ.

7   Paco Calvo, Vaidurya Sahi, and Anthony Trewavas, "Are Plants Sentient?" *Plant, Cell & Environment* 40, no. 11 (November 2017): 2858–2869, doi.org/10.1111/pce.13065.

8   Jennifer Frazer, "Dying Trees Can Send Food to Neighbors of Different Species," *Scientific American*, May 9, 2015, blogs.scientificamerican.com/artful-amoeba/dying-trees-can-send-food-to-neighbors-of-different-species.

9   Kat McGowan, "How Plants Secretly Talk to Each Other," *Wired*, December 20, 2013, www.wired.com/2013/12/secret-language-of-plants.

10 Brian Owens, "Trees Share Vital Goodies Through a Secret Underground Network," *NewScientist*, April 14, 2016, newscientist.com/article/2084488-trees-share-vital-goodies-through-a-secret-underground-network.

11 Bob Fischer and Andy Lamey, "Field Deaths in Plant Agriculture," *Journal of Agricultural and Environmental Ethics* 31, no. 4 (August 2018): 409–28, link.springer.com/article/10.1007/s10806-018-9733-8; Anna Hess and Mark Hamilton, "Calories Per Acre for Various Foods," *The Walden Effect* (blog), June 2010, www.waldeneffect.org/blog/Calories_per_acre_for_various_foods/.

12 "Children in the Fields Campaign," Association of Farmworker Opportunity Programs, accessed January 2, 2020, afop.org/cif/#tab-id-2.

13 Peter Whoriskey and Rachel Siegel, "Cocoa's Child Laborers," *Washington Post*, June 5, 2019, www.washingtonpost.com/graphics/2019/business/hershey-nestle-mars-chocolate-child-labor-west-africa/.

14 Estelle Higonnet, Marisa Bellantonio, and Glenn Hurowitz, "Chocolate's Dark Secret: How the Cocoa Industry Destroys National Parks," MightyEarth.org, September 12, 2017, www.mightyearth.org/wp-content/uploads/2017/09/chocolates_dark_secret_english_web.pdf

15 Steven L. Davis, "The Least Harm Principle May Require That Humans Consume a Diet Containing Large Herbivores, Not a Vegan Diet," *Journal of Agricultural and Environmental Ethics* 16, no. 4 (July 2003): 387–94, link.springer.com/article/10.1023/A:1025638030686.

CHAPTER 14: WHY DID MEAT BECOME TABOO?

1   Marta Zaraska, *Meathooked: The History and Science of Our 2.5-Million-Year Obsession with Meat* (New York: Basic Books, 2016).

2   "Chicken and Food Poisoning," Centers for Disease Control and Prevention, updated August 20, 2019, www.cdc.gov/foodsafety/chicken.html.

3   James Andrews, "CDC Shares Data on *E. Coli* and Salmonella in Beef," Food Safety News, October 29, 2014, www.foodsafetynews.com/2014/10/cdc-shares-mass-of-data-on-e-coli-and-salmonella-in-beef/.

4   Calvo, Sahi, and Trewavas, "Are Plants Sentient?"

5   Ellen G. White, "Chapter 23: Flesh Meats (Proteins Continued)," in *Counsels on Diet and Foods* (Washington, DC: Review and Herald, 1938), on the Ellen G. White Writings Website, accessed January 2, 2020, m.egwwritings.org/en/book/384.3093.

6   Stephen Nissenbaum, *Sex, Diet, and Debility in Jacksonian America* (Westport, CT: Prager, 1980).

7   "American College of Lifestyle Medicine Announces Dietary Lifestyle Position Statement for Treatment and Potential Reversal of Disease," PRWeb, September 25, 2018, www.prweb.com/releases/american_college_of_lifestyle_medicine_announces_dietary_lifestyle_position_statement_for_treatment_and_potential_reversal_of_disease/prweb15786205.htm.

8   Belinda Fettke, "Lifestyle Medicine . . . Where Did the Meat Go?," ISupportGary.com, November 28, 2018, isupportgary.com/articles/the-plant-based-diet-is-vegan and isupportgary.com/uploads/articles/ACLM-Presidents-Desk-LC-bashing.pdf.

9   Primetime Live, ABC News, July 30, 1992; Center for Consumer Freedom Team, "'PCRM Week': The AMA's Admonishments of PCRM," Center for Consumer Freedom, April 14, 2005, www.consumerfreedom.com/2005/04/2786-pcrm-week-the-amas-admonishments-of-pcrm/.

10 "Proof PETA Kills," Peta Kills Animals, a project of the Center for Consumer Freedom, accessed January 2, 2020, www.petakillsanimals.com/proof-peta-kills/#why-peta-kills and www.petakillsanimals.com/wp-content/uploads/2014/05/PetaKillsAnimals.pdf.

11 Vesanto Melina, Winston Craig, and Susan Levin, "Position of the Academy of Nutrition and Dietetics: Vegetarian Diets," *Journal of the Academy of Nutrition and Dietetics* 116, no. 12 (December 2016): 1970–80, www.eatrightpro.org/-/media/eatrightpro-files/practice/position-and-practice-papers/position-papers/vegetarian-diet.pdf.

12 Francesco Buscemi, "Edible Lies: How Nazi Propaganda Represented Meat to Demonise the Jews," *Media, War & Conflict* 9, no. 2 (2016), journals.sagepub.com/doi/abs/10.1177/1750635215618619.

13 Buscemi, "Edible Lies."

14 "Alexandra Jamieson: I'm Not Vegan Anymore," CBC Radio, May 15, 2013, www.cbc.ca/radio/thecurrent/may-15-2013-1.2909943/alexandra-jamieson-i-m-not-vegan-anymore-1.2909945; Erika Adams, "Vegan Blogger Ditches Veganism, Death Threats Ensue," Racked, July 10, 2014, www.racked.com/2014/7/10/7587289/vegan-blogger-receives-death-threats-after-eating-fish-and-eggs.

15 Cassidy Dawn Graves, "When Vegan Influencers Quit Being Vegan, the Backlash Can Be Brutal," Vice.com, August 29, 2019, www.vice.com/en_us/article/j5ymak/rawvana-vegan-youtube-influencers-quit-veganism.

16 "Farmers 'Sent Death Threats by Vegan Activists,'" BBC News, January 29, 2018, www.bbc.com/news/av/uk-42860384/farmers-sent-death-threats-by-vegan-activists; Livia Albeck-Ripka, "Protests in Australia Pit Vegans Against Farmers," *New York Times*, April 10, 2019, www.nytimes.com/2019/04/10/world/australia/vegans-protest-farms.html; Kate Larsen, "'I was feeling my life leave my body': Animal Rights Activist Says He Was Almost Killed While Protesting at a Petaluma Duck Farm," ABC7News.com, June 6, 2019, abc7news.com/activist-says-he-was-almost-killed-while-protesting-at-petaluma-duck-farm-/5334414/.

17 Nancy Matsumoto, "Sustainable Meat Supporters and Vegan Activists Both Claim Bullying," Civil Eats, January 10, 2017, nancymatsumoto.com/articles/2017/2/3/sustainable-meat-supporters-and-vegan-activists-both-claim-bullying.

18 Natalie Orenstein, "Local Butcher Shop Hangs Animal-Rights Sign Under Duress to Stop Protests," Berkeleyside Nosh, August 2, 2017, www.berkeleyside.com/2017/08/02/berkeleys-local-butcher-shop-hangs-animal-rights-sign-stop-weekly-protests; Lucy Pasha-Robinson, "Vegan Animal Rights Activists Are 'Sending Farmers Death Threats' Branding Them 'Murderers,'" Independent, January 29, 2018, www.independent.co.uk/news/uk/home-news/vegan-animal-rights-activists-farmers-death-threats-murderers-veganism-a8183091.html.

19 Eleanor Beardsley, "French Butchers Ask for Protection After Threats from Militant Vegans," The Salt (blog), NPR, July 18, 2018, www.npr.org/sections/thesalt/2018/07/18/628141545/french-butchers-ask-for-protection-after-threats-from-violent-vegans.

CHAPTER 15: WHY EAT ANIMALS IF WE COULD SURVIVE ON ONLY PLANTS?

1 Yanping Li et al., "Time Trends of Dietary and Lifestyle Factors and Their Potential Impact on Diabetes Burden in China," Diabetes Care 40, no. 12 (December 2017): 1685–94, care.diabetesjournals.org/content/40/12/1685.

2 "Fast-Food Restaurants and Industry in China–Market Research Report," IBISWorld, June 2019, www.ibisworld.com/industry-trends/international/china-market-research-reports/accommodation-catering/fast-food-restaurants.html.

3 Joseph Hincks, "The World Is Headed for a Food Security Crisis. Here's How We Can Avert It," Time, March 28, 2018, time.com/5216532/global-food-security-richard-deverell/.

4 Olga Gertcyk, "First-Ever Cases of Obesity in Arctic Peoples as Noodles Replace Traditional Diet," Siberian Times, February 20, 2017, siberiantimes.com/science/opinion/features/f0289-first-ever-cases-of-obesity-in-arctic-peoples-as-noodles-replace-traditional-diet/.

5 "Nunavik Food Guide Educator's Handbook," Nunavik Regional Board of Health and Social Services, accessed February 11, 2020, nrbhss.ca/sites/default/files/3.4.1.1_Educator%20handbook%20ENG.pdf.

6 Doris Gagné et al., "Traditional Food Consumption Is Associated with Higher Nutrient Intakes in Inuit Children Attending Childcare Centres in Nunavik," International Journal of Circumpolar Health 71 (2012), www.ncbi.nlm.nih.gov/pmc/articles/PMC3417681/.

CHAPTER 16: FEEDING THE WORLD

1 Paul Ausick, "When Does 'Too Much Oil' Become the Problem?," 24/7 Wall Street, October 21, 2016, 247wallst.com/energy-economy/2016/10/21/when-does-too-much-oil-become-the-problem/.

NOTES

2   Sarah Murray, "How Education Can Moderate Population Growth," World Economic Forum, July 27, 2015, www.weforum.org/agenda/2015/07/how-education-can -moderate-population-growth/.

3   Gerald Nelson et al., "Income Growth and Climate Change Effects on Global Nutrition Security to Mid-century," *Nature Sustainability* 1 (2018): 773–81, www. nature.com/articles/s41893-018-0192-z.epdf.

4   Gerald C. Nelson, "The Global Food Problem Isn't What You Think," *Washington Post*, January 2, 2019, www.washingtonpost.com/opinions/2019/01/02/ global-food-problem-isnt-what-you-think/.

5   Keiichiro Kanemoto et al., "Meat Consumption Does Not Explain Differences in Household Carbon Footprints in Japan," *One Earth* 1, no. 4 (December 2019): 464–71, www.cell.com/one-earth/fulltext/S2590-3322(19)30226-X.

6   Kathleen Gold, "Analysis: The Impact of Needle, Syringe, and Lancet Disposal on the Community," *Journal of Diabetes Science and Technology* 5, no. 4 (2011): www.ncbi. nlm.nih.gov/pmc/articles/PMC3192588/.

7   Monica Grafals and Ramon Sanchez, "The Environmental Impact of Dialysis vs Transplantation" (abstract), *American Journal of Transplantation* 16, no. S3 (2016), atcmeetingabstracts.com/abstract/the-environmental-impact-of-dialysis-vs -transplantation/.

8   Russell Knight, "Cattle & Beef Sector at a Glance," United States Department of Agriculture, updated August 28, 2019, www.ers.usda.gov/topics/animal-products/ cattle-beef/sector-at-a-glance.

9   "Range & Pasture," United States Department of Agriculture Natural Resources Conservation Service, accessed January 2, 2020, www.nrcs.usda.gov/wps/portal/nrcs/ main/national/landuse/rangepasture.

10 Office of the High Commissioner for Human Rights, "Venezuela: Dire Living Conditions Worsening by the Day, UN Human Rights Experts Warn," OHCHR. org, February 9, 2018, www.ohchr.org/en/NewsEvents/Pages/DisplayNews. aspx?NewsID=22646&LangID=E.

11 "Food Sovereignty," US Food Sovereignty Alliance, usfoodsovereigntyalliance.org/ what-is-food-sovereignty, accessed February 11, 2020.

INDEX

INDEX

PCRM (Physicians Committee for Responsible Medicine), 210–211, 212
Pearce, David, 193
People for the Ethical Treatment of Animals (PETA), 211
Peretti, Jacques, 18, 19
pet food industry, 31
PETA (People for the Ethical Treatment of Animals), 211
Physicians Committee for Responsible Medicine (PCRM), 210–211, 212
phytic acid, 95
pigs. *See* pork
plant proteins, 38. *See also* meat alternatives; plant-based diets; plants
    calories and, 61
    compared to animal protein, 38
    cost of, 81
    Nutrivore Challenge and, 253–254
    protein quality of, 87–92
plant-based diets. *See also* meat-free diets; plants; vegetarian/vegan diets
    climate and, 201
    deficiencies and, 219
    iron in, 95
    privilege and, 217–222
    ultraprocessed foods in, 91
    water usage and, 201
plants. *See also* cereals; grains; legumes; plant proteins; plant-based diets; soy
    antinutrients in, 94–95
    digestibility of, 96–97
    effects of producing, 115, 175, 176, 197–202. *See also* industrial row-crop agriculture
    ethics and, 206
    importance of, 97
    nutrients in, 92–93
    preparation of, 96–97
    protein equivalents in, 91
    raw, 97
    reasons to eat, 92–93
    satiation and, 61
    sentience and, 195–196, 206
    in traditional diets, 98
plowing, 143, 166
polarization, 214–216
policy. *See also* dietary guidelines; government; recommendations; subsidies
    Amazon fires, 170
    food aid policies, 237–238
    ideology and, 210–211
    obesity and, 237
    observational research and, 40–41
    regional reliance and, 237–238
    separation from research, 50–56
politics. *See also* government; policy

food insecurity and, 235–236
    polarization in, 214
pollutants, agrochemical, 10. *See also* fertilizers
Polyface Farms, 166, 168, 184
population
    carrying capacity of earth, 226–228
    food production and, 13
pork, 150, 154, 156
portion size, 49, 254
postdomestic society, 14
poultry. *See also* chicken; meat
    intake of, 32
    nutrients in, 71–72
    production of, 154–155
Poverty, Inc. (film), 238
precipitation, 161, 162. *See also* water
predators, 193, 199
pregnancy, vegetarian/vegan diet and, 105–106
prices of foods, 81–84
privilege. *See also* socioeconomic status
    ethics and, 184–185, 217–222
    vegetarian/vegan diet and, 97
processed foods, 14, 26, 55. *See also* hyperpalatable foods; junk food; ultraprocessed foods
    defined, 14
    health and, 220
    obesity and, 60
    in plant-based diets, 86
processed meats, 43, 57–58
profits, 132, 231, 235. *See also* economies, local
property rights, 228
protein. *See also* animal proteins; meat; plant proteins
    absorption of, 94
    access to/affordability of, 84
    appropriate intake of, 30, 32–38, 55
    dietary success and, 55
    health and, 36–37
    insufficient, 36–37
    satiation and, 60
protein digestibility-corrected amino acid score (PDCAAS), 87
protein equivalents, 90–91
protein-leverage hypothesis, 37
proteins, plant-based. *See* plant proteins

Q

Quebec, 221–222
questionnaires, 44–45, 110

R

rainfall, 161, 162. *See also* water
rainforest, 159, 170

INDEX

ABOUT THE AUTHORS

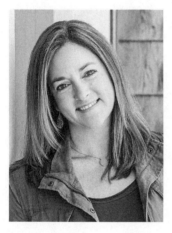

Photo © Joy Uyeno LeDuc

DIANA RODGERS, RD, is a "real food" nutritionist living on a working organic farm. She runs a clinical nutrition practice and speaks internationally about the intersection of optimal human nutrition and environmental sustainability. Diana is an advisory board member of Animal Welfare Approved, Savory Institute, and Whole30. She is also the producer of the *Sustainable Dish Podcast* and the director and producer of the film *Sacred Cow: The Case for Better Meat.* She can be found on social media @sustainabledish and on her two websites, Sustainabledish.com and Sacredcow.info.

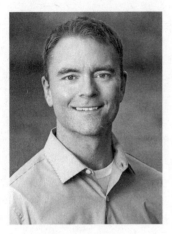

Photo © Neil Lockhard

ROBB WOLF is a former research bio-chemist and two-time *New York Times/WSJ* best-selling author. Robb has functioned as a review editor for the *Journal of Nutrition and Metabolism* (Biomed Central) and as a consultant for the Naval Special Warfare Resiliency program. He serves on the board of directors/advisers for: Specialty Health Inc, The Chickasaw Nation's "Unconquered Life" initiative, and a number of innovative start-ups with a focus on health and sustainability.